ADVANCE PRAISE FOR
Clinical Manual of Palliative Care Psychiatry

"**T**his is a clearly written and evidence-based book on psychiatry in palliative care. Reading this book will go a long way to helping specialist palliative care clinicians feel comfortable dealing with psychiatric illnesses. A must read!"

> —**Robert Arnold, M.D.**, Leo H. Criep Chair in Patient Care, Chief Medical Officer, UPMC Palliative and Supportive Institute, University of Pittsburgh

"**W**ith the imperative that psychiatry fully embrace its role among other medical specialties in the management of complex illness, the psychiatric literature is enhanced by timely publications which enhance models of multispecialty care. Drs. Fairman, Hirst, and Irwin have produced a tightly organized, succinct, pragmatic, and current clinical handbook on palliative care psychiatry that is an important contribution to the field. Effectively bridging the relevant areas of psychosomatic medicine and geriatric psychiatry, they show how the consultation psychiatrist is a critical member of the multispecialty and multidisciplinary teams treating patients in a palliative care model. Their chapters cover the critical areas of clinical palliative care psychiatry practice, with especially thoughtfully written chapters on delirium, dementia, insomnia, pain management, substance use disorders, psychotherapy, and the palliative care of children. Their use of tables and figures to illustrate their approach to palliative care patients is especially well done. This book will be of great value to psychosomatic medicine and geriatric psychiatrists, but is equally highly recommended for the general psychiatrist and child and adolescent psychiatrist who will need to care for critically and terminally ill patients as well."

> —**James A. Bourgeois, O.D., M.D.**, Clinical Professor and Vice Chair, Clinical Affairs, Department of Psychiatry/Langley Porter Psychiatric Institute, University of California, San Francisco

"**P**sychiatry is a very valuable but underutilized resource in oncology, palliative care, geriatrics, and long-term care. The frequency of serious psychological concerns is quite high in those with advanced illness, and this book is a unique resource that addresses all aspects of suffering and effective treatment. This comprehensive resource on how psychiatry can enhance palliative care should be required reading for all professionals working with the seriously ill and dying."

> —**Stephen R. Connor, Ph.D.** [...]ative Care Alliance (WHPCA)

"Comprehensive! Concise! Practical! Packed with useful information. The guide I have been waiting for to assist psychiatric residents, psychosocial oncology teams, and oncologists in the practice of primary palliative care. Added bonuses are the tables and the additional resources at the back of each chapter. This manual is a must-read for every clinician dealing with advanced illness and end-of-life issues."

—**Mary Helen Davis, M.D., DFAPA,** Integrative Psychiatry, Behavioral Oncology and Palliative Care Consultant; Associate Clinical Professor of Psychiatry, University of Louisville School of Medicine, Kentucky

"Drs. Fairman, Hirst, and Irwin's new book, *Clinical Manual of Palliative Care Psychiatry,* is a critically important contribution to this evolving specialty known as palliative care psychiatry. The 11 chapters are comprehensive yet concise, with excellent tables; several chapters are devoted to specific psychiatric complications which practitioners regularly encounter in their clinical work with patients with life-limiting illnesses. Consultation-liaison psychiatry services will find this volume essential for both trainees and senior clinicians who are caring for patients at the end of life."

—**Jon A. Levenson, M.D.,** Associate Professor of Psychiatry, Columbia University Medical Center; Attending Psychiatrist, Division of Consultation-Liaison Psychiatry; Director, Undergraduate Medical Education in Consultation-Liaison Psychiatry

"The *Clinical Manual of Palliative Care Psychiatry* is a concise and clearly written handbook that will be useful to psychiatric physicians, advance practice nurses, and other professionals working at the bedside of patients with serious illness. Intuitively organized, its brief and helpful chapters provide the newcomer with critical overviews, and the more experienced clinician with a framework to be sure he/she has hit all the marks. Fairman, Hirst, and Irwin have done a commendable job of condensing the most up-to-date evidence into a pocket-type guide that should inform and improve clinical care for years to come."

—**Thomas B. Strouse, M.D., FAPM, DFAPA,** Maddie Katz Professor of Palliative Care Research and Education; Vice-Chair for Clinical Affairs, UCLA David Geffen School of Medicine Department of Psychiatry

"The content of the *Clinical Manual* is extraordinarily expert, well structured, and well presented. The clearly written text, figures, and tables all provide critically important information to the psychiatric and palliative care clinician, enabling her/him to rapidly enhance her/his knowledge, clinical judgment, and clinical care delivery."

—**Deane L. Wolcott, M.D., DLFAPA, FAPM, FAPOS,** Director, Oncology Supportive Care Services, Samuel Oschin Comprehensive Cancer Institute, Cedars-Sinai Medical Center, Los Angeles, California

"Well-referenced, easy-to-use, and clinically practical, the *Clinical Manual of Palliative Care Psychiatry* skillfully addresses some of the most challenging aspects of palliative medicine. This book should be in every hospice and palliative medicine physician's library, as well as every psychiatrist who cares for this important patient population. Drs. Fairman, Hirst, and Irwin are leading experts in palliative care psychiatry, and I am thrilled that they have shared their wisdom with us to the benefit of all our patients."

—**Holly Yang, M.D., M.S.H.P.Ed., HMDC, FAAHPM, FACP,** Scripps Health, San Diego, California

Clinical Manual of Palliative Care Psychiatry

Clinical Manual of Palliative Care Psychiatry

By

Nathan Fairman, M.D., M.P.H.
Assistant Clinical Professor,
Department of Psychiatry and Behavioral Sciences
University of California Davis School of Medicine
Sacramento, California

Jeremy M. Hirst, M.D.
Associate Clinical Professor, Department of Psychiatry;
Associate Director, Palliative Care Psychiatry;
Associate Director, Patient and Family Support Services,
Moores Cancer Center
University of California San Diego School of Medicine
La Jolla, California

Scott A. Irwin, M.D., Ph.D.
Associate Professor of Psychiatry;
Director, Supportive Care Services,
Samuel Oschin Comprehensive Cancer Institute
Cedars-Sinai Medical Center
Los Angeles, California

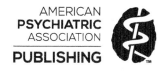

AMERICAN
PSYCHIATRIC
ASSOCIATION
PUBLISHING

If you wish to buy 50 or more copies of the same title, please go to www.appi.org/specialdiscounts for more information.

Copyright © 2016 American Psychiatric Association Publishing
ALL RIGHTS RESERVED
Manufactured in the United States of America on acid-free paper
20 19 18 17 16   5 4 3 2 1
First Edition
Typeset in Adobe Garamond Pro and Helvetica LT.

American Psychiatric Association Publishing
1000 Wilson Boulevard
Arlington, VA 22209-3901
www.appi.org

Library of Congress Cataloging-in-Publication Data
Names: Fairman, Nathan, 1972– , author. | Hirst, Jeremy M., author. | Irwin, Scott A., author. | American Psychiatric Association Publishing, publisher.
Title: Clinical manual of palliative care psychiatry / by Nathan Fairman, Jeremy M. Hirst, Scott A. Irwin.
Description: First edition. | Arlington, Virginia : American Psychiatric Association Publishing, [2016] | Includes bibliographical references and index.
Identifiers: LCCN 2016000325 (print) | LCCN 2016000910 (ebook) | ISBN 9781585624768 (pbk. : alk. paper) | ISBN 9781615370610 ()
Subjects: | MESH: Palliative Care—psychology | Psychiatry—methods | Terminally Ill—psychology | Psychotherapy
Classification: LCC RT87.T45 (print) | LCC RT87.T45 (ebook) | NLM WB 310 | DDC 616.02/9—dc23
LC record available at http://lccn.loc.gov/2016000325

British Library Cataloguing in Publication Data
A CIP record is available from the British Library.

To our families, friends, colleagues, mentors, and patients:
You have had more impact on us than you can ever know,
and we are in your debt.

Contents

PART I
Background and Context

PART II
Core Clinical Applications

PART III
Other Common Psychiatric Conditions

List of Tables

List of Figures

Foreword

When I first took care of a patient with a terminal illness complicated by psychiatric problems, in a hospice unit in a large urban teaching hospital in Chicago around 1989, I asked for a consultation from the hospital's consultation-liaison psychiatry service. The psychiatrist came, saw the patient, left the room, and said, "She's dying. Who could cope with that?" and walked away, never to return. The message to me as an internal medicine resident was not to consult psychiatrists for help with sick patients—they are useless. Instead, I learned what I would call "first-line" psychiatry as part of being an internist—taking to heart the admonition that 70% of internal medicine practice is psychiatric anyway. When I have been mistaken for a psychiatrist (because I listen to patients talk), I have always been quick to say, "Oh, noooo, I'm not a psychiatrist! I'm taking care of sick people, helping them cope with a serious illness—that's part of 'normal' medicine!"

Along the road to my own specialization in the new field of hospice and palliative medicine, I met a few psychiatrists who were clinically helpful—but they were notable for their rarity. One feature of their rarity was that they were not afraid of taking care of patients who were really sick. I would goad psychiatrists with the observation that the *Diagnostic and Statistical Manual of Mental Disorders,* the bible of psychiatric diagnosis, opened with the caveat that no psychiatric diagnosis could be made in a patient who had a serious illness, yet those were the very patients for whom I needed help. These rare individuals would say, "Yes, I know, that's why it's so difficult. Now how can I help you with your patient?" I would characterize this small group as outliers, much like the early pioneers in hospice and palliative medicine, who often seemed not to "fit in" with the rest of medicine. Secretly, I wished that I could work regularly with such an individual.

Later in life, my wish was granted. Not only did I have the pleasure of working with Dr. Scott Irwin in a large hospice inpatient unit and large home hospice practice, but he attracted others. Dr. Jeremy Hirst and Dr. Nathan Fairman came to train with Dr. Irwin, and then to practice in the hospice and palliative medicine environment, including the affiliated cancer center and children's hospital. My reaction, and that of the 26 other physicians and 8 nurse practitioners in our group, was something like, "We had no idea how much we were missing and how useful these psychiatrists can be for the patients, their families, we providers, and the nurses, social workers, and chaplains on our interdisciplinary teams."

Now, many years later, I am of the opinion that any group specializing in palliative medicine needs the "right" psychiatrist as a partner—someone willing to join in taking care of the patients, looking after the emotional and psychological experience of being really sick, and teaching the group members his or her helpful approaches to working with these patients. This psychiatrist practicing in palliative care would say that this is a new subspecialty in the practice of psychiatry. I believe it.

This book is meant to help disseminate that knowledge so that more suffering can be relieved and more quality of life preserved, restored, and sustained. From my own experience and that of my patients and colleagues, when this information is made practically available, the clinical outcomes are always better and are sometimes miraculous. It gives me great professional satisfaction to see this book published, and to see the interest not only of psychiatrists but also of other clinicians in making this information their own—for the benefit of their patients and families and the staff working with them.

I am of the opinion that many of the challenges of contemporary practice can be traced to the mind-body dualism that was a product of philosopher René Descartes's bargain with the Roman Catholic Church during the Enlightenment. Modern medicine suffers from giving the body to most of the doctors and reserving the mind for the psychiatrists. If I were king, I would make psychiatry one of the principal specialties of medicine—right alongside cardiology, nephrology, and oncology. I'd bring the neurologists right along with them. It is all the medicine of human beings—whole persons with physical, emotional, practical, and spiritual dimensions that need to be considered together in health and illness. This book brings us closer to that goal. The more each of us tries to learn about people in all of their delightful complexity, the better clinicians we will be.

Charles F. von Gunten, M.D., Ph.D., F.A.C.P., F.A.A.H.P.M.
Vice President, Medical Affairs, Hospice and Palliative Medicine,
OhioHealth, Columbus, Ohio

Introduction

It was true, as the doctor said, that Ivan Ilych's physical sufferings were terrible, but worse than the physical sufferings were his mental sufferings, which were his chief torture.

Leo Tolstoy, *The Death of Ivan Ilych*

Context and Audience

Perhaps it goes without saying that individuals with serious medical illness, particularly as they approach the very end of life, often experience significant psychological distress. As referenced in the epigraph above, Leo Tolstoy made this observation in the late 1800s in his famous novella, *The Death of Ivan Ilych,* identifying "mental sufferings" as Ivan Ilych's "chief torture." More recently, Cicely Saunders, the English physician credited with establishing the tenets of modern hospice care, observed that in patients with advanced cancer, "mental distress may be perhaps the most intractable pain of all." Hence, it should come as no surprise that the psychological dimensions of suffering in seriously ill patients warrant expert attention as part of the comprehensive, person-centered approach that typifies palliative care.

Nonetheless, in our experience—as psychiatrists practicing in inpatient palliative care and home-based hospice clinical settings—we have routinely encountered a gulf between principles and practice when it comes to providing skillful mental health care in palliative care settings. It is not uncommon for us to work with clinicians on both sides of this divide: on one side, the front-line palliative care providers who lack formal mental health training yet are eager to improve their ability to address psychiatric symptoms, and on the other side, mental health specialists who lack familiarity with palliative care yet are eager to improve their effectiveness in participating with palliative care clinicians in the care of seriously ill and dying patients. This book is aimed at helping to bridge that gap, by addressing the needs of both groups.

This book can be positioned alongside other efforts to develop an interface between psychiatry and palliative care. Much of the content of palliative care psychiatry has been recorded in a comprehensive text, Chochinov and Breitbart's *Handbook of Psychiatry in Palliative Medicine,* first published in 2000 and now in its second edition (published in 2009 by Oxford University Press). Newer developments, in several different domains, have helped to refine and expand this body of knowledge. This work has included, for example, research on the rapid treatment of depression in seriously ill patients, practice guidelines for the management of terminal delirium, and the new psychotherapies developed specifically for patients nearing the very end of life. Taken together, these and other contributions embody a subspecialty field at the intersection of palliative care and psychiatry, an emerging discipline that brings expertise in understanding the psychosocial dimensions of human experience to the care of seriously ill patients and the support of their families.

Content and Organization

The book begins with a review of the basic tenets and practice models of palliative care (Chapter 1), followed by an overview of opportunities for psychiatric involvement in the care of seriously ill patients in palliative care settings (Chapter 2). Shifting focus to the bedside, the book then offers a focused, practical approach to treatment of three of the most commonly encountered psychiatric conditions in palliative care: depression, anxiety, and delirium (Chapters 3–5). Dementia and insomnia are addressed next (Chapters 6 and 7). Substance use disorders can greatly complicate the management of patients with advanced medical disease, as explored in Chapter 8. Several psychotherapies, reviewed in Chapter 9, have recently been developed specifically for the palliative care setting. Chapter 10 provides an overview of pain management, followed by a review of psychotropic medications used as adjuvant analgesic drugs. Finally, Chapter 11 covers special considerations in the psychiatric care of children and adolescents with serious illness.

Content in each chapter emphasizes the features of assessment and management that are unique to the setting of palliative care. In addition, each chapter concludes with a list of supplemental materials aimed at directing readers to relevant content that may be of interest. Specifically, additional resources include relevant chapters from the Chochinov and Breitbart text (providing a broader conceptual base and historical context), Fast Facts from the Center to Advance Palliative Care (providing a practical, succinct treatment of specific clinical issues), links to relevant modules from the Education in Palliative and End-of-Life Care curriculum, and other pertinent books, papers, or online resources.

Caveats

Readers should be aware of several caveats regarding this book. First, as an emerging field of practice, palliative care psychiatry has very few studies of the highest quality design on which to base clinical decision making. Concerns about generalizability can be raised about most research informing the practice of psychiatric palliative care. In general, the approaches to assessment and treatment that are described in this book are based on a combination of data extrapolated from general clinical populations, expert opinion, and practice-based experience.

Second, as a corollary, readers should be aware that drug treatments in palliative care—including many of those described in this text—often involve off-label medication use. In practice, readers should consult the most current references, make use of consultation with local experts, and be certain to explicitly discuss with patients the basis for medication recommendations in the clinical setting.

Third, in developing a text that intends to be focused and clinically relevant, certain trade-offs with regard to breadth and depth are necessary. This text, for example, does not cover the management of challenging personalities, or approaches to supporting caregivers around issues of grief and bereavement. Similarly, there is a set of common ethical issues that frequently arise in the palliative care setting, and a psychiatrist's expertise can often be beneficial in helping clinicians, patients, and families develop acceptable solutions in such situations. These issues, however, are beyond the scope of this book, and interested readers are encouraged to find guidance for these topics from other resources.

Conclusion

We expect that readers drawn to this book will already have some motivation to improve their skills in the psychiatric care of seriously ill patients—whether they are seasoned palliative care experts wanting to hone their ability to address psychological dimensions of suffering, or experienced mental health specialists seeking to contribute more effectively to the interdisciplinary approach to care in a palliative care setting.

We hope that readers will find motivation in this book to help push the field of palliative care psychiatry further forward. As alluded to in this introduction (and described in more detail in Chapter 2, "Psychiatry in Palliative Care"), this book draws from and builds on the work of many others in helping to improve the psychiatric care of patients with serious illnesses. There remains a great need for novel research, education, and systems-level interventions to help further develop the field of palliative care psychiatry.

Finally, our ultimate hope is that this book will be helpful in empowering clinicians to more skillfully respond to "mental sufferings" in seriously ill and dying patients.

Nathan Fairman, M.D., M.P.H.
Jeremy M. Hirst, M.D.
Scott A. Irwin, M.D., Ph.D.

Disclosure of Competing Interests

The authors had no competing interests during the year preceding manuscript submission.

PART I

Background and Context

Palliative Care 101

This chapter provides an overview of the —development of palliative care as a model for providing care to individuals with complex, advanced medical illness. The core tenets of palliative care practice are reviewed, as are some of the benefits of palliative care.

Definitions: Palliative Care and Hospice

Several definitions of *palliative care* appear in the medical literature and in materials from professional societies. The existence of different definitions has probably contributed to misconceptions and low levels of awareness about palliative care. In public opinion polling in 2011, for example, 70% of adults described themselves as "not at all knowledgeable" about palliative care (Center to Advance Palliative Care 2011). Similarly, even among physicians, low levels of knowledge and misinformed attitudes have sometimes contributed to misperceptions about palliative care (Brickner et al. 2004; Hanratty et al. 2006; Ogle et al. 2002).

Two of the most widely cited definitions of *palliative care* are provided in Table 1–1. The World Health Organization's definition captures the core fea-

3

Table 1–1.   Definitions of palliative care

World Health Organization	Center to Advance Palliative Care
Palliative care improves the quality of life of patients and families who face life-threatening illness, by providing pain and symptom relief, spiritual and psychosocial support from diagnosis to the end of life and bereavement. Palliative care • Provides relief from pain and other distressing symptoms; • Affirms life and regards dying as a normal process; • Intends neither to hasten nor postpone death; • Integrates the psychological and spiritual aspects of patient care; • Offers a support system to help patients live as actively as possible until death; • Offers a support system to help the family cope during the patient's illness and in their own bereavement; • Uses a team approach to address the needs of patients and their families, including bereavement counseling, if indicated; • Will enhance quality of life, and may also positively influence the course of illness; and • Is applicable early in the course of illness, in conjunction with other therapies that are intended to prolong life, such as chemotherapy or radiation therapy, and includes those investigations needed to better understand and manage distressing clinical complications. (World Health Organization 2015)	Palliative care, also known as palliative medicine, is specialized medical care for people living with serious illness. It focuses on providing relief from the symptoms and stress of a serious illness—whatever the diagnosis. The goal is to improve quality of life for both the patient and the family. Palliative care is provided by a team of palliative care doctors, nurses and other specialists who work together with a patient's other doctors to provide an extra layer of support. It is appropriate at any age and at any stage in a serious illness and can be provided along with curative treatment. (Center to Advance Palliative Care 2011)

tures of the discipline: "Palliative care improves the quality of life of patients and families who face life-threatening illness, by providing pain and symptom relief, spiritual and psychosocial support from diagnosis to the end of life and bereavement" (World Health Organization 2015). Some of the most important—and often misunderstood—elements of palliative care include a focus on preserving quality of life, attention to varied sources of distress in both the patient and caregivers, reliance on a team with interdisciplinary expertise, and use of interventions that complement disease-oriented treatments throughout the entire course of an illness. Also, particularly relevant to mental health specialists, definitions of palliative care explicitly acknowledge the need to attend to psychological dimensions of suffering, as part of a comprehensive whole-person and family-oriented approach to care.

A further distinction will help to clarify the nature of palliative care, which is both a general approach to care and a medical subspecialty. As shown in Table 1–2, palliative care exists along a continuum from primary to tertiary levels of expertise. All clinicians involved in caring for seriously ill patients should have basic competencies in providing primary palliative care, whereas clinicians with specialist-level training can provide the secondary and tertiary levels of palliative care that are needed for more challenging cases (Quill and Abernethy 2013; von Gunten 2012). For physicians, specialist-level expertise is obtained through fellowship training in hospice and palliative medicine, a subspecialty medical field formally recognized in 2006. (The term *palliative medicine* generally refers to the physician subspecialty, whereas *palliative care* refers to the broader approach to patient care, delivered by an interdisciplinary team of specialists.) The subspecialty is sponsored by 10 medical boards, including the American Board of Psychiatry and Neurology, and training involves completion of a 1-year postgraduate fellowship. Similarly, specialist-level certification programs exist for palliative care nursing, social work, and chaplaincy.

Finally, *hospice* is a particular model of specialized palliative care. Hospice services can be provided when the prognosis is short and the goals of therapy are to optimize quality of life and support patients and families as life comes to an end. In the United States, hospice services are generally available to individuals with a prognosis of 6 months or less, and services are largely governed by the guidelines of the federal Medicare hospice benefit.

Table 1–2.   Three levels of palliative care expertise

Primary palliative care

All clinicians

Attention to whole person and family concerns

Attention to symptom burden and quality of life

Treatment rooted in understanding of individual's unique illness experience

Basic clarification of goals of therapy

Knowledge of when specialist consultation is needed

Secondary palliative care

Specialists (physician, registered nurse, social worker, chaplain, etc.)

Interdisciplinary, team-based care (e.g., hospice program, palliative care consultation service)

Tertiary palliative care

Care provided in major referral centers (e.g., academic hospital)

Specialists (physician, registered nurse, social worker, chaplain, etc.)

Interdisciplinary, team-based care (e.g., hospice program, palliative care consultation service)

Care for the most challenging cases

Leadership in research and education

Training of others in primary and secondary palliative care

Source.   Adapted from Quill and Abernethy 2013 and von Gunten 2012.

Basic Tenets of Palliative Care

Total Pain

The English physician Cicely Saunders is widely credited with establishing modern standards of hospice care though her work with cancer patients in London in the mid-1900s. Conceptually, her seminal contribution was to articulate the concept of *total pain,* which posits that dying patients experience pain in physical, emotional, spiritual, and practical dimensions. With this all-encompassing concept of pain, Saunders advocated for a more person-centered and comprehensive approach to care at the end of life, one that sought to address not only the nociceptive components of a patient's pain but also—and just as important—the emotional, spiritual, and experiential dimensions of suffering. As a consequence, careful attention to addressing total pain remains one of the central tenets of contemporary palliative care (Clark 1999).

Others have operationalized Saunders's conception of total pain. From the standpoint of identifying the roles for mental health expertise in palliative care, the model advanced by Ferris et al. (2002) is particularly useful. As illustrated in Figure 1–1, this model delineates eight dimensions of distress commonly experienced by seriously ill patients and their families. Hence, the concept of total pain is embodied in the interdisciplinary approach to patient care that characterizes modern-day palliative care, in which a team with varied expertise (nurses, social workers, chaplains, physicians, etc.) is essential to the success of identifying and addressing the various dimensions of suffering.

Person-Centered, Goal-Driven Care

Beyond the concept of total pain, other core features of palliative care practice, shown in Table 1–3, include the following: 1) organizing care around the needs of patients and their families, 2) utilizing a team with interdisciplinary expertise to identify and address the various dimensions of suffering, 3) clarifying achievable goals of care, and 4) structuring interventions in time-limited therapeutic trials with clearly articulated clinical targets.

In palliative care, the term *goals of care* is used to refer to the broad aims of medical therapy, in relation to each patient's values and preferences, taking into account the patient's particular medical situation. In the setting of advanced, serious illness, patients and their families have a wide range of goals with respect to their medical disease: some hope for a cure, many hope for prolongation of life, and all hope for relief from the multiple issues that contribute to their suffering (Ferris et al. 2002). Ideally, medical care is aimed at enabling patients to achieve goals that are closely aligned with their values and preferences. Hence, patient and family goals provide the foundation for patient-centered and family-oriented care.

Clarifying goals often involves a process of mutual education: the physician provides information about the medical context, the appropriate medical in-

Disease Management

Primary diagnosis,
   prognosis, evidence
Secondary diagnoses (e.g.,
   dementia, psychiatric
   diagnoses, substance use,
   trauma)
Comorbidities (e.g.,
   delirium, seizures, organ
   failure)
Adverse events (e.g., side
   effects, toxicity)
Allergies

Physical

Pain and other symptoms[a]
Level of consciousness,
   cognition
Function, safety, aids:
   Motor (e.g., mobility,
   swallowing, excretion)
   Senses (e.g., hearing,
   sight, smell, taste,
   touch)
   Physiological (e.g.,
   breathing, circulation)
   Sexual
Fluids, nutrition
Wounds
Habits (e.g., alcohol,
   smoking)

Psychological

Personality, strengths,
   behavior, motivation
Depression, anxiety
Emotions (e.g., anger,
   distress, hopelessness,
   loneliness)
Fears (e.g., abandonment,
   burden, death)
Control, dignity,
   independence
Conflict, guilt, stress, coping
   responses
Self-image, self-esteem

Loss, Grief

Loss
Grief (e.g., acute, chronic,
   anticipatory)
Bereavement planning
Mourning

**Patient and Family
Characteristics**

Demographics (e.g., age,
   gender, race, contact
   information)
Culture (e.g., ethnicity,
   language, cuisine)
Personal values, beliefs,
   practices, strengths
Developmental state,
   education, literacy
Disabilities

Social

Cultural values, beliefs,
   practices
Relationships, roles
   with family, friends,
   community
Isolation, abandonment,
   reconciliation
Safe, comforting
   environment
Privacy, intimacy
Routines, rituals, recreation,
   vocation
Financial resources,
   expenses
Legal (e.g., powers of
   attorney for business,
   for healthcare, advance
   directives, last will/
   testament, beneficiaries)
Family caregiver protection
Guardianship, custody
   issues

**End-Of-Life Care/
Death Management**

Life closure (e.g.,
   completing business,
   closing relationships,
   saying goodbye)
Gift giving (e.g., things,
   money, organs, thoughts)
Legacy creation
Preparation for expected
   death
Anticipation and
   management of
   physiological changes
   in the last hours of life
Rites, rituals
Pronouncement,
   certification
Perideath care of family,
   handling of the body
Funerals, memorial services,
   celebrations

Practical

Activities of daily living (e.g.,
   personal care, household
   activities, …)[b]
Caregiving
Dependents, pets
Telephone access,
   transportation

Spiritual

Meaning, value
Existential, transcendental
Values, beliefs, practices,
   affiliations
Spiritual advisors, rites,
   rituals
Symbols, icons

Figure 1–1.   Dimensions of distress in advanced, life-limiting illness *(opposite page).*

[a]Other common symptoms include (but are not limited to) the following: **Cardiorespiratory:** breathlessness, cough, edema, hiccups, apnea, agonal breathing patterns; **Gastrointestinal:** nausea, vomiting, constipation, obstipation, bowel obstruction, diarrhea, bloating, dysphagia, dyspepsia; **Oral:** dry mouth, mucositis; **Dermal:** dry skin, nodules, pruritus, rashes; **General:** agitation, anorexia, cachexia, fatigue, weakness, bleeding, drowsiness, effusions (pleural, peritoneal), fever/chills, incontinence, insomnia, lymphedema, myoclonus, odor, prolapse, sweats, syncope, vertigo.

[b]Examples of personal care include ambulation, bathing, toileting, feeding, dressing, and transfers. Examples of household activities include cooking, cleaning, laundry, banking, and shopping.

Source.   Reprinted from Ferris FD, Balfour HM, Bowen K, et al.: "A Model to Guide Patient and Family Care: Based on Nationally Accepted Principles and Norms of Practice." *Journal of Pain and Symptom Management* 24(2):106–123, 2002. Used with permission.

Table 1–3.   Basic tenets of palliative care practice

Person-centered and family-oriented care	Interventions are driven by the needs of patient and family.
Domains of distress and interdisciplinary expertise	Care is provided by a diverse team of specialists who assess and addresses various dimensions of distress.
Clarifying goals of care	Patients and families are assisted in articulating broad, achievable goals, framed in terms of their values and preferences; therapies are aligned to those goals.
Time-limited therapeutic trials	Interventions are structured with clear clinical targets and end points, with regular assessment of outcomes.

terventions, and the range of achievable clinical outcomes, framed in terms that are understandable and meaningful to the patient, whereas the patient educates the physician about his or her values and preferences, and about what things matter most to him or her within the context of the illness experience and disease trajectory. In addition, because patients and families sometimes have overlapping or conflicting goals of care, a conversation that clarifies goals often includes a discussion about potential trade-offs that may be encountered as clinicians try to bring treatments into alignment with multiple goals. (For example, treatments aimed at the goal of alleviating pain may undermine the goal of preserving mentation; in such a case, the patient would need to help the clinician understand how he or she would make trade-offs between those two important goals.) Once goals have been clarified, patients, family members, and clinicians often have a clearer understanding of which particular interventions will be most consistent with the patient's goals. Goals often evolve over time, as a disease progresses and other changes develop in patients' lives; hence, the clarification of goals is also an iterative, dynamic process, and revisiting goals as the disease evolves is central to the provision of person-centered care.

Benefits of Palliative Care

Palliative care has been shown to provide enhanced value through its effects on both quality and cost. Table 1–4 provides an overview of selected research findings supporting the benefits of palliative care. In terms of quality measures, numerous studies, from diverse practice settings and using a wide variety of study design, have shown improvements in symptom control, self-reported quality of life, and satisfaction of patients and caregivers (Teno et al. 2004; Yennurajalingam et al. 2011). Newer studies have begun to suggest that early palliative care interventions confer a survival benefit in some conditions (Temel et al. 2010). Similarly, in terms of measures of cost and resource allocation, there is solid evidence that many models of palliative care can help to contain costs and provide efficiencies in resource allocation, often through minimizing the provision of unwanted therapies (Kelley et al. 2013; Morrison et al. 2011; Norton et al. 2007).

Table 1–4.   Selected evidence for the benefits of palliative care

Measures	Results	Study description
Quality measures		
Symptom control	Reduced pain, fatigue, dyspnea, insomnia, depression, anxiety (Yennurajalingam et al. 2011)	Retrospective analysis of more than 400 cancer patients receiving outpatient palliative care
Quality of life	Improved subjective quality of life (Yennurajalingam et al. 2011)	Retrospective analysis of more than 400 cancer patients receiving outpatient palliative care
Patient and caregiver satisfaction	Higher levels of emotional support, greater perception of having been treated with respect, higher assessment of quality of care (Teno et al. 2004)	Nationally representative sample of family members of deceased patients who used home-based hospice services (vs. matched control subjects)
Survival	Increased survival in metastatic lung cancer: Patients receiving palliative care plus standard cancer therapy lived approximately 2.5 months longer (Temel et al. 2010)	Randomized controlled trial of standard cancer care vs. standard cancer care plus outpatient palliative care in adults with metastatic non-small-cell lung cancer at time of diagnosis

Table 1–4.   Selected evidence for the benefits of palliative care (*continued*)

Measures	Results	Study description
Cost measures		
Resource use	Reduced intensive care unit length of stay (Norton et al. 2007)	Small prospective pre/postperformance study of the effect of inpatient palliative care consultation
	Reduced total costs per admission (Morrison et al. 2011)	Study of influence of inpatient palliative care consultation in Medicaid beneficiaries at four acute care hospitals in New York State
	Reduced cost of care at end of life (Kelley et al. 2013)	Longitudinal survey of nationally representative cohort of older adults; hospice enrollees vs. non-hospice matched control subjects

---

Conclusions and Key Points

- *Palliative care* refers to a model of care designed for patients with complex, serious medical illnesses, which aims to preserve quality of life and alleviate distress, in both the patient and loved ones, throughout the entire course of an illness.

- Palliative care is provided along a continuum, from the primary palliative care of the generalist to the secondary and tertiary palliative care delivered by specialist practitioners.

- The core tenets of palliative care include attention to the dimensions of distress (total pain), provision of care by a multispecialty and multiprofessional team, clarification of patient and family goals and alignment of treatment with those goals, and use of time-limited therapeutic trials.

- The benefits of palliative care include improvements in quality of care (symptom control, quality of life, satisfaction, survival) and reductions in cost and resource utilization.

References

Brickner L, Scannell K, Marquet S, et al: Barriers to hospice care and referrals: survey of physicians' knowledge, attitudes, and perceptions in a health maintenance organization. J Palliat Med 7(3):411–418, 2004 15265350

Center to Advance Palliative Care: Public opinion research on palliative care. 2011. Available at: http://www.capc.org/tools-for-palliative-care-programs/marketing/public-opinion-research/2011-public-opinion-research-on-palliative-care.pdf. Accessed July 18, 2015.

Clark D: "Total pain," disciplinary power and the body in the work of Cicely Saunders, 1958–1967. Soc Sci Med 49(6):727–736, 1999 10459885

Ferris FD, Balfour HM, Bowen K, et al: A model to guide patient and family care: based on nationally accepted principles and norms of practice. J Pain Symptom Manage 24(2):106–123, 2002 12231127

Hanratty B, Hibbert D, Mair F, et al: Doctors' understanding of palliative care. Palliat Med 20(5):493–497, 2006 16903402

Kelley AS, Deb P, Du Q, et al: Hospice enrollment saves money for Medicare and improves care quality across a number of different lengths-of-stay. Health Aff (Millwood) 32(3):552–561, 2013 23459735

Morrison RS, Dietrich J, Ladwig S, et al: Palliative care consultation teams cut hospital costs for Medicaid beneficiaries. Health Aff (Millwood) 30(3):454–463, 2011 21383364

Norton SA, Hogan LA, Holloway RG, et al: Proactive palliative care in the medical intensive care unit: effects on length of stay for selected high-risk patients. Crit Care Med 35(6):1530–1535, 2007 17452930

Ogle KS, Mavis B, Wyatt GK: Physicians and hospice care: attitudes, knowledge, and referrals. J Palliat Med 5(1):85–92, 2002 11839230

Quill TE, Abernethy AP: Generalist plus specialist palliative care—creating a more sustainable model. N Engl J Med 368(13):1173–1175, 2013 23465068

Temel JS, Greer JA, Muzikansky A, et al: Early palliative care for patients with metastatic non-small-cell lung cancer. N Engl J Med 363(8):733–742, 2010 20818875

Teno JM, Clarridge BR, Casey V, et al: Family perspectives on end-of-life care at the last place of care. JAMA 291(1):88–93, 2004 14709580

von Gunten CF: Evolution and effectiveness of palliative care. Am J Geriatr Psychiatry 20(4):291–297, 2012 22367161

World Health Organization: WHO definition of palliative care. 2015. Available at: http://www.who.int/cancer/palliative/definition/en/. Accessed June 18, 2015.

Yennurajalingam S, Urbauer DL, Casper KL, et al: Impact of a palliative care consultation team on cancer-related symptoms in advanced cancer patients referred to an outpatient supportive care clinic. J Pain Symptom Manage 41(1):49–56, 2011 20739141

Additional Resources

American Academy of Hospice and Palliative Medicine. Web site at: http://aahpm.org.

Center to Advance Palliative Care. Web site at: http://www.capc.org.

Du Boulay S: Cicely Saunders: The Founder of the Modern Hospice Movement. London, Ashford Color Press, 2007

Dy S, Grant M. UNIPAC 4: The Hospice and Palliative Care Approach to Serious Illness. UNIPAC Self Study Program, 4th Edition. Edited by Storey CP Jr. Glenview, IL, American Academy of Hospice and Palliative Medicine 2012. Available at: http://

www.aahpm.org/resources/default/unipac-4th-edition.html. Accessed July 16, 2015.

Hanks G, Cherny NI, Christakis NA, et al (eds): Oxford Textbook of Palliative Medicine, 4th Edition. New York, Oxford University Press, 2009

Shuster JL, Higginson IJ: Hospice and palliative care: a psychiatric perspective, in Handbook of Psychiatry in Palliative Medicine, 2nd Edition. Edited by Chochinov HM, Breitbart W. New York, Oxford University Press, 2009, pp 3–12

Palliative Care Subspecialty Certification

Physician: American Academy of Hospice and Palliative Medicine. Web site at: http://aahpm.org/career/.

Nursing: National Board for Certification of Hospice and Palliative Nurses. Web site at: https://www.nbchpn.org/DisplayPage.aspx?Title=RN%20Overview.

Social Work: National Association of Social Workers. Web site at: http://www.socialworkers.org/credentials/credentials/achp.asp.

Chaplaincy: Board of Chaplaincy Certification. Web site at: http://bcci.professionalchaplains.org/content.asp?contentid=42.

2

Psychiatry in Palliative Care

Chapter Overview

This chapter focuses on the emergence of a field of clinical expertise at the interface of psychiatry and palliative care. Following a brief historical perspective on psychological considerations in the care of patients with complex medical illness, there is a review of several areas in which psychiatric palliative care has recently evolved. The chapter closes with an overview of opportunities and roles for psychiatry within palliative care, setting the stage for subsequent chapters that pursue these topics in greater detail.

Historical Perspective: Psychological Considerations in Palliative Care

Serious psychological and emotional symptoms frequently accompany a life-threatening illness, and the psychiatric dimensions of suffering have been an area of focus in palliative care since the earliest stages of the development of the field. Cicely Saunders, for example, describing the management of cancer pain, once observed that "mental distress may be perhaps the most intractable pain of all" (Saunders 1963, p. 197). The World Health Organization's (2015) definition of palliative care (provided in full in Table 1–1 in Chapter 1, "Palliative Care 101") also makes specific reference to this important component of treatment: "Palliative care...integrates the psychological and spiritual aspects of patient care."

Despite their shared awareness that seriously ill patients and their families often experience significant psychological distress, early models of hospice and palliative care seldom included psychiatrists. Several barriers to psychiatric involvement have been described (Billings and Block 2009; Meier and Beresford 2010). Some impediments relate to professional factors, such as the belief among palliative care providers that they themselves could adequately address psychological distress, or the lack of confidence among psychiatrists about their ability to be of value in caring for patients near the end of life. Practice patterns within the field of psychiatry may have hindered the field's involvement as well, because the emergence of palliative care coincided with a movement in psychiatry toward increasing reliance on psychopharmacology and away from psychotherapeutic modes of care. Systems-level factors, including funding structures that have been unfamiliar or inadequate to compensate psychiatry providers, may also have been barriers.

Emergence and Evolution of Palliative Care Psychiatry

Despite the barriers just mentioned, recent progress has been made in expanding the interface between psychiatry and palliative medicine. Over the past decade, the field of palliative care has matured in many concrete ways—for example, through increased utilization of hospice services, with the establishment of palliative medicine as a formally recognized medical subspecialty, and through opportunities for advanced certification of palliative care consultation services via The Joint Commission. Similarly, in the same time period, psychiatrists and other mental health specialists have increasingly found ways to bring their expert skills and knowledge to the care of seriously ill patients, even as they near the final phase of life. Hence, palliative care psychiatry, which shares overlap with psychosomatic medicine and psycho-oncology, may be understood as an emerging subspecialty discipline at the intersection of palliative medicine and psychiatry (Fairman and Irwin 2013; Irwin and Ferris 2008).

Much of the conceptual content of palliative care psychiatry has been captured in a text, *Handbook of Psychiatry in Palliative Medicine,* now in its second edition (Chochinov and Breitbart 2009). This body of knowledge continues to be enlarged and refined by important new data from clinical research in many different domains (Fairman and Irwin 2013).

Palliative care psychiatry is also embodied in the small group of psychiatrists now certified as subspecialists in hospice and palliative medicine—another indicator of psychiatric involvement in subspecialty-level palliative care. The hospice and palliative medicine certification examination has been administered four times, in 2008, 2010, 2012, and 2014, and the numbers of passing examinees sponsored by the American Board of Psychiatry and Neurology were 15, 12, 34, and 0, respectively[1] (J. Vollmer, personal communication, January 20, 2015).

Yet another indication of the emergence of palliative care psychiatry—tracking the growth of palliative care more broadly—is the high level of interest among psychiatry trainees in educational experiences focused on palliative care. Irwin et al. (2011) provided data from a survey of general psychiatry training directors and residents, revealing that formal learning opportunities around palliative care psychiatry are lacking, despite a high degree of interest among trainees. These authors also reported that a rotation in psychiatric palliative care (involving supervised clinical experiences in a community-based hospice program, communication training, and didactic instruction in core palliative care content) was associated with significant improvements in competence and knowledge, as well as reduced apprehension about practicing in the palliative care setting.

The evolution of palliative care psychiatry has occurred in several different practice models. For example, one major community-based nonprofit hospice established an in-house psychiatry program to provide access to specialist-level expertise in addressing the emotional distress of hospice patients and their caregivers (American Psychiatric Association 2009). Also, a small number of

---

[1] The 2012 examination represented the last opportunity for clinicians to qualify for the subspecialty under the practice pathway, and all subsequent examinees are required to have completed an accredited fellowship in hospice and palliative medicine. In 2014, 2.4% of all examinees were sponsored by the American Board of Psychiatry and Neurology, but none of those passed the exam.

academic centers in the United States now include psychiatrists on their palliative care teams, frequently in leadership roles (Meier and Beresford 2010). Other models have been developed abroad. In Japan, for example, cancer hospitals receiving funding support through the federal insurance program are required to include a psychiatrist on interdisciplinary palliative care teams. Ogawa et al. (2012) reported improvements in access to psychiatric consultation and treatment services among hospitals with palliative care teams that met this federal requirement to include psychiatrists.

Opportunities for Psychiatry in Palliative Care

Where, exactly, do psychiatrists fit into palliative care? What roles can they play? How can psychiatric expertise improve the care of patients in palliative care settings? The Ferris et al. (2002) model of the dimensions of distress (see Figure 1–1 in Chapter 1) is particularly useful in helping to identify opportunities for psychiatric involvement in palliative care. Even setting aside the obvious psychological dimension—wherein many patients struggle with depression, anxiety, or other significant psychological symptoms—nearly all the other domains include important areas in which a psychiatrist may contribute unique expertise in palliation (Irwin and Ferris 2008). Table 2–1 lists some of the potential sources of suffering in advanced medical illness that may benefit from psychiatric expertise. Psychiatrists may contribute, for example, by advising drug treatments for the management of neuropathic pain; by facilitating the process of life closure (e.g., through supporting intimacy in relationships near the end of life); and by helping to address concerns about bereavement. Furthermore, effective management of psychosocial and psychiatric issues often enables improvements in other domains, as evidenced, for example, by the reduction in physical pain that frequently follows effective treatment of depression.

Table 2–2 lists some of the areas of psychiatric expertise that can enhance palliative care. Above all else, the psychiatrist's diagnostic expertise is essential in beginning to alleviate psychological distress. In the setting of serious, advancing medical illness, distinguishing among normal sadness, grief, adjustment disorder, and major depression, as one example, can be quite challenging. Similarly, anxiety, delirium, dementia, and other psychiatric syndromes are

Table 2–1.   Sources of suffering in advanced medical illness that may benefit from psychiatric expertise

Abandonment	Distress
Anger	Fear
Anxiety	Grief
Bereavement	Hope/hopelessness
Boundary-setting	Insomnia
Burden	Loneliness
Caregiving	Loss
Coping	Nausea
Delirium	Pain
Dementia	Personality issues
Denial	Professional burnout/self-care
Dependence	Shortness of breath
Depression	Substance use problems
Desire for hastened death	Suicidal ideation
Dignity	

Source.   Reprinted from Irwin SA, Ferris FD: "The Opportunity for Psychiatry in Palliative Care." *Canadian Journal of Psychiatry* 53(11):713–724, 2008. Used with permission.

common in palliative care settings and are frequently underrecognized or underappreciated, although they can contribute substantially to the burden of suffering for patients and families. These conditions may be present as comorbidities, or they may result from the natural progression of disease. Similarly, they could represent expressions of difficulty with coping or adverse effects of treatment. The process of untangling and differentiating among possible psychiatric diagnoses and medical causes of psychiatric symptoms—so that appropriate interventions can be provided—often requires the involvement of an experienced psychiatrist (Block 2006; Irwin and Ferris 2008).

Table 2–2.   Roles for psychiatric expertise in palliative care

Providing diagnostic expertise

Providing expertise in treatment planning:

- Psychopharmacological interventions (especially off-label uses)
- Nonpharmacological interventions
- Psychotherapies

Clarifying ethical concerns (e.g., through the assessment of decisional capacity)

Providing education about psychiatric palliative care:

- To front-line clinicians
- To trainees (in many disciplines)

Caring for the family (e.g., addressing issues of loss and bereavement)

Assisting with challenging communication tasks

Supporting clinicians with issues of self-care and burnout

Developing research efforts aimed at improving patient care

The psychiatrist can also provide expertise in treatment planning, including the use of medication, nonpharmacological interventions, and psychotherapies. Expertise in psychopharmacology, in addition to enhancing patient care, often unburdens nonpsychiatric providers from practicing beyond their comfort level. For example, treating depression near the end of life frequently includes the careful use of psychostimulants, a strategy that is often outside the experience of generalist providers. Similarly, because the management of anxiety and agitation frequently involves off-label use of psychotropic medication, expertise in psychopharmacology is vitally important.

Expert-level knowledge and skills of psychotherapy can complement or broaden the therapeutic skills of other members of the palliative care team. Although all providers can combine skillful communication and a compassionate presence in providing basic psychotherapy at the bedside, and many providers will have more advanced skills in supportive psychotherapy approaches, the mental health specialist brings the skill set of an expert and the ability to use specific psychotherapy approaches that have been developed for or adapted to the palliative care setting.

The use of nonpharmacological strategies may be vital as well, particularly with respect to challenging psychiatric conditions for which medication interventions can involve significant risks. The psychiatrist's expertise can help to ensure that nonpharmacological approaches are optimized, for example, in the management of agitated behavior in dementia or delirium.

Finally, other roles for psychiatrists in palliative care may include educating front-line clinicians about psychiatric distress, or helping clinicians in addressing issues of loss and bereavement in seriously ill patients. Palliative care providers experience their own grief as well, and the psychiatrist can often help teams with debriefing complex and challenging cases, and with supporting self-care and grief responses. Additionally, palliative care psychiatrists can often help to clarify ethical questions, such as through the assessment of capacity (especially when an affective disturbance or cognitive deficit is felt to cloud the judgment of a patient making complex medical decisions). As the field continues to move forward, palliative care psychiatrists will have important opportunities to contribute to the education of trainees (in many disciplines) and to the continued expansion of clinical research focused on issues specific to psychiatric palliative care (Fairman and Irwin 2013).

Conclusions and Key Points

- Patients with serious, advanced illnesses frequently experience symptoms that benefit from psychiatric expertise.

- Palliative care psychiatry represents an emerging field at the interface of palliative care and psychiatry.

- Psychiatrists familiar with the basic tenets of palliative care can make important contributions to the care of seriously ill patients and their loved ones.

References

American Psychiatric Association: Integrating mental health services into hospice settings: the Palliative Care Psychiatric Program, San Diego Hospice and the Institute for Palliative Medicine, San Diego. Psychiatr Serv 60(10):1395–1397, 2009 19797386

Billings JA, Block SD: Integrating psychiatry and palliative medicine: the challenges and opportunities, in Handbook of Psychiatry in Palliative Medicine, 2nd Edition. Edited by Chochinov HM, Breitbart W. New York, Oxford University Press, 2009, pp 13–20

Block SD: Psychological issues in end-of-life care. J Palliat Med 9(3):751–772, 2006 16752981

Chochinov HM, Breitbart W (eds): Handbook of Psychiatry in Palliative Medicine, 2nd Edition. New York, Oxford University Press, 2009

Fairman N, Irwin SA: Palliative care psychiatry: update on an emerging dimension of psychiatric practice. Curr Psychiatry Rep 15(7):374, 2013 23794027

Ferris FD, Balfour HM, Bowen K, et al: A model to guide patient and family care: based on nationally accepted principles and norms of practice. J Pain Symptom Manage 24(2):106–123, 2002 12231127

Irwin SA, Ferris FD: The opportunity for psychiatry in palliative care. Can J Psychiatry 53(11):713–724, 2008 19087465

Irwin SA, Montross LP, Bhat RG, et al: Psychiatry resident education in palliative care: opportunities, desired training, and outcomes of a targeted educational intervention. Psychosomatics 52(6):530–536, 2011 22054622

Meier DE, Beresford L: Growing the interface between palliative medicine and psychiatry. J Palliat Med 13(7):803–806, 2010 20636148

Ogawa A, Nouno J, Shirai Y, et al: Availability of psychiatric consultation-liaison services as an integral component of palliative care programs at Japanese cancer hospitals. Jpn J Clin Oncol 42(1):42–52, 2012 22131342

Saunders C: The treatment of intractable pain in terminal cancer. Proc R Soc Med 56:195–197, 1963 13986816

World Health Organization: WHO definition of palliative care. 2015. Available at: http://www.who.int/cancer/palliative/definition/en/. Accessed June 18, 2015.

Additional Resources

Billings AJ, Block SD: Integrating psychiatry and palliative medicine: the challenges and opportunities, in Handbook of Psychiatry in Palliative Medicine, 2nd Edition. Edited by Chochinov HM, Breitbart W: New York, Oxford University Press, 2009, pp 13–20

Macleod AD: Palliative medicine and psychiatry. J Palliat Med 16:340–341, 2013

Meier DE, Beresford L: Growing the interface between palliative medicine and psychiatry. J Palliat Med 13:803–806, 2010

Strouse T: Palliative medicine and psychiatry: a reply. J Palliat Med 16:1166–1167, 2013

PART II

Core Clinical Applications

3

Depression

Chapter Overview

This chapter reviews the approach to addressing symptoms of depression in the palliative care setting. Such symptoms are common among individuals with advanced medical illness, and they range along a continuum from normal states of sadness to serious and debilitating symptoms seen in major depression. Significant symptoms of depression can greatly amplify the suffering of patients and their loved ones. Because several different conditions can be marked by depressed mood, this chapter provides guidance in distinguishing among these different conditions in the palliative care setting. Even among seriously ill patients, and even near the very end of life, major depression can often be effectively addressed; therefore, management strategies—including both psychosocial interventions and pharmacological treatments—are reviewed here, with particular emphasis on the unique aspects of management in the palliative care setting.

Feelings of depression are common among seriously ill patients, and such symptoms exist on a continuum, ranging from the transient feelings of sadness that are a normal part of the human condition to the unrelenting and debilitating impairments in mood and cognition that are experienced in major depressive disorder. Unfortunately, among patients with advanced medical illnesses, clinicians and caregivers often overlook the impact of psychological symptoms such as depression because they assume that these are normal or expected experiences. However, prompt and effective management of depression is an important therapeutic aim because, even among patients with an advanced medical illness, various interventions are available that can ameliorate depression, thereby reducing suffering and improving quality of life. As such, there is a great need for competency in the identification, diagnosis, and management of depression in palliative care settings.

Epidemiology and Consequences

Epidemiology

Estimates for the prevalence of depression in palliative care settings range widely, depending on the definitions used and populations studied. Nonetheless, most data suggest that both symptoms of depression and depressive disorders are present at higher levels among palliative care populations than among healthy individuals. For example, major depression occurs in approximately 7% of the general population (American Psychiatric Association 2013), but data suggest that the disorder affects 13.1% of patients with advanced cancer (Wilson et al. 2007). Similarly, major depressive disorder appears to be present in about 14.3%–16.5% of patients in palliative care settings, depending on the criteria used for diagnosis (Mitchell et al. 2011).

Consequences

When unrecognized or inadequately treated, depression can be associated with significant morbidity and mortality. High levels of psychological distress can negatively impact physical health and quality of life, complicate the management of a primary illness, and contribute to significant distress in the patient, loved ones, and clinicians (Hirdes et al. 2012; Wilson et al. 2009). In addition to being a well-known risk factor for suicide in general populations, depression in patients with advanced medical illness is associated with the desire for hastened death (Breitbart et al. 2000; Chochinov et al. 1995; Rodin et al. 2009; Rosenfeld et al. 2014), and it influences the will to live in cancer patients receiving palliative care (Chochinov et al. 1999). Increasingly, depression has been recognized as a powerful factor influencing disease progression and mortality in cancer (Giese-Davis et al. 2011; Spiegel 2011). In one meta-analysis focused on patients with cancer, for example, minor or major depression was associated with a 39% increased risk of death, and depressive symptoms were associated with a 25% increased risk of death, after adjustment for a variety of factors, suggesting that depression may independently influence mortality in patients with cancer (Satin et al. 2009).

Symptoms, Screening, and Differential Diagnosis

Symptoms

Symptoms of depression may present as obvious changes in mood (feeling sad, down, blue, deflated, etc.) or as an inability to experience pleasure in previously enjoyable activities. In the setting of an advanced illness, such changes may be accompanied by disengagement from loved ones or apathy and low motivation to participate in treatment. Additionally, clinical depression is often associated with a variety of other symptoms, in behavioral, cognitive, and somatic domains, as described in the subsection "Differential Diagnosis" below. The emergence of any of these changes should raise suspicion for depression.

Many different conditions can contribute to symptoms of depression; these include, for example, physical exhaustion, uncontrolled pain, medications, physiological derangements, or concerns about being a burden to others. Table 3–1 lists some of the possible etiologies of depressive symptoms, as well as risk factors for depressive disorders. Strategies to treat symptoms of depression should begin with attempts to identify and address these conditions.

As with most other psychiatric illnesses, disorders of depression are established based on a *clinical diagnosis*. Although some screening tools (described in the next subsection, "Screening") can be helpful in identifying patients at risk for depression, there are no tests to establish a definitive diagnosis. In-

Table 3–1.   Etiologies, indicators, and risk factors for depression

Psychiatric causes

  Major depression

  Adjustment disorders

Medical causes

  Poorly controlled physical symptoms (e.g., pain, nausea, dyspnea, fatigue)

  Drugs (e.g., opioids, corticosteroids, benzodiazepines)

  Tumor involvement of central nervous system

  Infections (e.g., Epstein-Barr virus)

  Metabolic disturbances (e.g., abnormal levels of sodium or calcium)

  Nutritional problems (e.g., anemia or deficiencies in vitamin B_{12} or folate)

  Endocrine disorders (e.g., hypothyroidism or adrenal insufficiency)

  Neurological disorders (e.g., Parkinson's disease)

Psychological, social, and spiritual causes

  Grief

  Existential distress

  Concerns about family distress

  Overwhelming financial or family distress

  Hopelessness and meaninglessness

  Guilt

  Fear of expressing anger

  Sleep deprivation

Table 3–1.   Etiologies, indicators, and risk factors for
depression *(continued)*

Psychological indicators

Feelings of worthlessness

Excessive feelings of guilt

Anhedonia

Wishing for death

Feelings of hopelessness and helplessness

Suicidal ideation

Somatic signs and symptoms

Less valuable when assessing depression in seriously ill patients; the medical
illness itself can produce symptoms of fatigue, loss of energy, anorexia, and
insomnia

Risk factors

Family history of depression

History of affective disorder or alcohol use disorder

Advanced stage of illness

Increased physical impairment

Left hemispheric strokes

Pancreatic, breast, and lung cancers

Brain metastases

Younger age with advanced illness

Spiritual pain

Poor social support

Previous suicide attempts

Source.   Modified from Irwin SA, Fairman N, Montross LP: *UNIPAC 2: Alleviating Psychological and Spiritual Pain. UNIPAC Self Study Program,* 4th Edition. Edited by Storey CP Jr. Glenview, IL, American Academy of Hospice and Palliative Medicine, 2012. Used with permission.

stead, diagnosis relies on the subjective history of the patient, collateral information, and careful clinical observation—informed by knowledge of the risk factors for depression and the characteristics that distinguish the different conditions marked by depression.

Screening

Several simple, clinically useful screening instruments have been shown to improve the detection of depression. The Patient Health Questionnaire (Kroenke et al. 2001), the Hospital Anxiety and Depression Scale (Mitchell et al. 2010), and the Center for Epidemiologic Studies Depression Scale, Boston short form (Kohout et al. 1993) are perhaps the most widely used, and useful, instruments for identifying depressive states and/or monitoring severity of symptoms. However, their performance characteristics in the palliative care setting have not been systematically examined (Wasteson et al. 2009). Nonetheless, some data suggest that even the simple query "Are you depressed?" may have high validity in identifying depression in patients with terminal illness (Chochinov et al. 1997).

Differential Diagnosis: Major Depression and Its Look-Alikes

In seriously ill patients with symptoms of depression, one of the most challenging tasks is to distinguish among the many different conditions that are characterized by depression, ranging from normal sadness to major depression, and including a variety of conditions in between. Accurate characterization of these different entities is important because management strategies differ depending on the etiology and classification of symptoms. To take a common example, hypothyroidism may masquerade as depression, and the effective approach to alleviating symptoms would involve treating the underlying medical cause. Other psychiatric conditions, such as adjustment disorder, grief, and demoralization syndrome, need to be distinguished from major depression; the cardinal features of these conditions are summarized in Table 3–2 and described in detail below.

Table 3–2.   Psychiatric differential diagnoses for "depression"

Condition	Characteristics	General approach to treatment
Major depressive disorder	A. Five or more of the following present, over at least 2 weeks, and at least one of the symptoms is either depressed mood or anhedonia: 1. Depressed mood (or irritable mood in children or adolescents) 2. Anhedonia (i.e., markedly reduced interest or pleasure in most activities) 3. Changes in weight or appetite 4. Insomnia or hypersomnia 5. Psychomotor agitation or retardation 6. Fatigue or diminished energy 7. Feelings of worthlessness or excessive guilt 8. Poor concentration, or indecisiveness 9. Recurrent thoughts of death, suicidal ideation, or suicidal behavior B. Symptoms cause clinically significant distress or functional impairment.	Drug therapy + psychotherapy

Table 3–2.   Psychiatric differential diagnoses for "depression" (*continued*)

Condition	Characteristics	General approach to treatment
Major depressive disorder (*continued*)	C. Symptoms are not the result of substances or a medical condition. D. Symptoms are not better explained by one of the psychotic disorders. E. The patient has never experienced mania or hypomania.	
Unspecified depressive disorder	Clinically significant distress from depression, accompanied by functional impairment, but which does not meet criteria for any of the more specific depressive illnesses. **Note:** This diagnosis should not be used for patients experiencing normal sadness without clear functional consequences.	Continued assessment and clarification of diagnosis + psychotherapy
Adjustment disorder with depressed mood	Emotional or behavioral symptoms that develop within 3 months of an identifiable stressor. Symptoms are disproportionate to the severity or intensity of the stressor. May occur with features of depression, anxiety, behavior, or any combination. **Note:** If criteria are met for major depression, then major depression should be diagnosed and not adjustment disorder.	Supportive counseling aimed at bolstering resilience and coping skills Problem solving aimed at resolving or removing stressor

Table 3–2.   Psychiatric differential diagnoses for "depression" (continued)

Condition	Characteristics	General approach to treatment
Grief	In grief, the predominant emotional state is characterized by emptiness and loss; in major depression, it is depressed mood and/or inability to experience pleasure.	Supportive counseling or psychotherapy
	In grief, dysphoria often occurs in waves, generally triggered by thoughts or memories of the deceased; in major depression, dysphoria is unrelenting, and cognitions center on worthlessness or hopelessness.	
	In grief, the mood state is reactive (i.e., individuals can have periods of happiness, laughter, etc., in relation to pleasant or humorous experiences); in major depression, the mood state can be pervasive or intractable.	
	In grief, self-esteem may be preserved, and if feelings of guilt are present they are usually constrained to the relationship with the deceased.	
	In grief, thoughts of death often concern "joining" the deceased; in major depression, they are aimed at ending one's own life and rooted in feelings of hopelessness and worthlessness.	

Table 3–2.   Psychiatric differential diagnoses for "depression" (continued)

Condition	Characteristics	General approach to treatment
Grief (continued)	**Note:** Bereavement is no longer an exclusion criterion for major depression. Even in the setting of bereavement, if criteria are met for major depression, then major depression should be diagnosed and appropriate treatment initiated.	
Demoralization	Marked by subjective incompetence (perceived inability to make progress), hopelessness, despair, loss of meaning or purpose.	Supportive counseling or psychotherapy
	Often reactivity of mood is preserved.	
	Often develops in protracted serious illness with prolonged hospitalization.	
	Insufficient evidence for demoralization as a separate diagnostic category.	

Note.   Descriptions of disorders based on DSM-5 (American Psychiatric Association 2013). Description of demoralization based on Kissane et al. (2001) and Robinsor et al. (2016).

Source.   Modified from Fairman N, Hirst JM, Irwin SA: "Depression and Anxiety: Assessment and Management in Hospitalized Patients With Serious Illness," in *Hospital-Based Palliative Medicine: A Practical, Evidence-Based Approach.* Edited by Pantilar SZ, Anderson W, Gonzales M, et al. Hoboken, NJ, Wiley, 2015, pp. 71–91. Used with permission.

Major depressive disorder is the condition against which others are compared.[1] The hallmark of the disorder is the presence of a major depressive episode,[2] which is characterized by either a depressed mood or anhedonia (loss of
interest in pleasurable activity), occurring nearly every day, over a period of at
least 2 weeks.[3] Patients with major depressive disorder also experience a number of cognitive or somatic symptoms. Cognitive changes can include poor
concentration or indecision, and thoughts of worthlessness, hopelessness,
guilt, or death. Somatic symptoms can include changes in appetite or weight,
changes in sleep, decreased energy, or changes in psychomotor activity. As with
all psychiatric illnesses, significant functional impairment—major problems in
relationships, at work, or in self-care—needs to be present in order for the condition to be considered a disorder (American Psychiatric Association 2013).

As alluded to above, differentiating among the conditions marked by depression—and even separating these from the experience of normal sadness—
can often be quite challenging in palliative care settings, even for experienced
clinicians. It is not uncommon for seriously ill patients to experience intense
sadness; many endure periods of anhedonia, low motivation, and even hopelessness; and some may also contemplate death. However, none of these phenomena *alone* indicates the presence of major depression. Similarly, the
somatic dimensions of major depression (e.g., changes in sleep, low energy,
changes in weight and appetite) frequently overlap with the physical symptoms
seen in advanced medical illnesses (or resulting from their treatment), so these
are often not reliable indicators of major depression in this population. Instead,
experts in palliative care psychiatry give greater weight to the emotional and
cognitive symptoms of clinical depression, as well as changes in mood from
baseline, and the intensity and time course of symptoms (Block 2001). Thus,

---

[1] In this chapter, as well as in clinical practice in palliative care psychiatry, the terms *major depressive disorder, clinical depression,* and *major depression* are used interchangeably.
[2] A major depressive episode may be seen in bipolar disorder as well, and screening for
the absence of historical periods of mania or hypomania will distinguish major depressive disorder from bipolar disorder. This distinction is important therapeutically, because antidepressant therapy is less likely to be effective, and may even be harmful, in
depressed patients with bipolar illness.
[3] If neither depressed mood nor anhedonia is present, major depressive disorder should
not be diagnosed; other conditions need to be considered.

feelings of worthlessness, hopelessness, guilt, or thoughts of suicide point more strongly toward major depression. Similarly, the presence of *true anhedonia*—in which the patient has lost the ability to experience pleasure in previously enjoyable activities (and has not simply lost the ability to engage in those activities due to functional limitations)—helps to identify major depression. Usually, unless major depression is present, the ability to experience pleasure or joy (e.g., in the company of loved ones) is preserved, even when physical limitations preclude the ability to engage in enjoyable activities. On the other hand, changes in appetite or level of energy are more likely to be attributed to the underlying medical illness or side effects of treatment.

Although major depression is the illness that most clinicians have in mind when they refer to a patient as being "clinically depressed," several other important conditions may overlap with or be mistaken for major depressive disorder (see Table 3–2). Adjustment disorder results from an identifiable stressor, which causes marked distress (in the form of symptoms of depression, anxiety, or behavioral disturbances) to a degree in excess of the intensity of the stressor and without meeting criteria for a depressive or anxiety disorder. Often, adjustment disorders are most effectively addressed with nonpharmacological management strategies aimed at resolving or removing the stressor or bolstering resilience and coping skills.

Grief, the emotional experience associated with a significant loss, is also a distinct experience from major depression, although the two conditions have in common the experience of a depressed mood (Jacobsen et al. 2010). Of note, in the most recent edition of the *Diagnostic and Statistical Manual of Mental Disorders* (DSM-5), the "bereavement exception" was removed from the diagnosis of major depressive disorder, so that even in the setting of bereavement, major depression should be diagnosed (and treatment considered) if criteria are met (American Psychiatric Association 2013). This distinction is important, because the general approach to addressing grief (in the absence of major depression) should rely on supportive therapeutic interventions and not drug therapy, although medication for specific symptoms, such as insomnia, can be helpful for brief periods.

Demoralization syndrome includes a suite of psychological phenomena commonly seen in patients with advanced medical disease, which may overlap with major depression (Kissane et al. 2001). The condition is marked by hopelessness, helplessness, meaninglessness, and existential distress (Kissane et al.

2001; Robinson et al. 2016). A hallmark of demoralization, "subjective incompetence" refers to a patient's internal sense of ineptitude with respect to being able to make improvements, arising from the loss of purpose and meaning that can occur in a serious medical illness. Hence, in major depression, progress toward improvement is hindered by problems with motivation and drive, whereas in demoralization, improvement is undermined by a profound sense of incompetence and hopelessness about the possibility of improvement. Also, unlike depressed patients, the demoralized patient can generally experience happiness in relation to positive events (i.e., reactivity of mood). There is considerable debate, beyond the scope of this chapter, as to whether or not demoralization syndrome can be reliably distinguished from major depression and what interventions might be most appropriate. Nonpharmacological interventions generally should be given priority.

Additionally, two common neurocognitive disorders, delirium and dementia, may also sometimes be mistaken for depression, particularly when marked by social withdrawal, psychomotor retardation, and diminished motivation (see Chapter 5, "Delirium," and Chapter 6, "Dementia [Major Neurocognitive Disorder]"). In both conditions, the predominant symptom is a significant cognitive disturbance, with an onset that is generally insidious (in the case of dementia) or acute or subacute (in the case of delirium). Although cognitive deficits can occur in major depression, they tend to arise only after the emergence of changes in mood or the development of anhedonia, and they are often less severe than in primary neurocognitive disorders.

Management of Depression in the Palliative Care Setting

The general approach to addressing depression in seriously ill patients should be rooted in basic principles of palliative care: interventions ought to be informed by knowledge of prognosis and goals of care, optimal care is delivered by an interdisciplinary team, physical symptoms and other dimensions of distress need to be assessed and addressed, nonpharmacological interventions should be optimized, and pharmacological treatments should be provided in the context of time-limited goal-oriented trials.

As discussed in Chapter 1, "Palliative Care 101," the term *goals of care* refers to the aims of medical therapy in relation to the patient's values and preferences. Ideally, medical care is broadly aimed at enabling patients to achieve the goals that matter most to them, given the circumstances of their particular medical situation and other constraints. With respect to the management of depression in palliative care, knowledge of goals is important because the broad aims of therapy can inform choices about workup and intervention. Some patients and families, hoping for restoration to a previous level of quality of life, will pursue a workup and time-limited therapeutic trials aimed at reversal of the depression. For them, simple tests, such as a blood draw to investigate for hypothyroidism, may be acceptable, especially if the results might help to identify a therapeutic intervention (e.g., thyroid hormone replacement) that could alleviate the "depression" and thereby improve quality of life. For others, ensuring comfort and dignity may be higher priorities, and therefore care may focus instead on avoiding burdensome testing, managing distressing symptoms, and providing measures aimed purely at the relief of suffering. In some situations, antidepressants might be acceptable for these goals, whereas in other situations, the thought of taking another pill is just too burdensome or the risk is too great. Also, in some cases, a goals clarification may uncover preferences about management that are influenced by stigma or prior experience with mental health treatment, which ought to be sensitively explored with the patient and family as part of the process of developing a care plan for depression.

Fully informed decision making in this setting requires a thorough discussion of the medical situation (including the expected prognosis, likely etiology of depressive symptoms, and risks and burdens associated with potential interventions), *complemented by* an explication of the patient's goals under the circumstances. In the setting of depression, this process can sometimes be particularly challenging, because a patient's decisions (and capacity for autonomous decision making) may be influenced by the depression itself.

Management strategies differ depending on the etiology and classification of symptoms (the general approach to treatment for different depressive conditions is summarized in Table 3–2). For major depressive disorder, the "gold standard" treatment includes a combination of patient and family education, psychotherapy, and antidepressant medication. Other modalities (complementary and alternative therapies) have also been proposed for the management of depression, although limited data are available specific to their impact on ameliorating depression in palliative care settings. Nonetheless, a substantial body of high-quality evidence supports the efficacy of combined treatment with psychotherapy and medication, and these approaches can be employed in addressing depression in the palliative care setting (Block and ACP-ASIM End-of-Life Care Consensus Panel 2000).[4] Figure 3–1 provides an overview of the general approach to managing depression in palliative care settings.

Patient and Family Education

Providing education to the patient and family can include a clear discussion of the diagnostic assessment (and its rationale), review of treatment options and the associated risks and benefits, and efforts to address stigma. These efforts are supported by current practice guidelines (Gelenberg et al. 2010), and they may help to promote adherence to treatment, improve response to therapy, and improve psychosocial functioning in adults with depression (Tursi et al. 2013). In the palliative care setting, patient and family education dovetails with clarification of goals, as noted in the earlier subsection "Management of Depression in the Palliative Care Setting."

Psychotherapy

Importantly, even the busiest clinician can provide valuable psychosocial support at the bedside. Some of the most basic elements of establishing rapport—use of active listening skills, seeking to understand patients' concerns, engaging loved ones, and mobilizing support systems—will go a long way toward reducing distress in depressed patients. Formal psychotherapy interventions, often arranged through consultation with therapists with expertise in the care of medically ill patients, should be considered for any patient with high levels of psychological distress, irrespective of the etiology. There is moderate-quality evidence that a variety of psychotherapies can be effective in treating depressive symptoms in palliative care settings, but no single intervention has been found to be more effective than others (Li et al. 2012). Among the ther-

---

[4]Electroconvulsive therapy (ECT) is also a highly effective treatment for depression, particularly suited for geriatric patients or for patients with treatment-resistant depression, serious medical illness, and a prognosis of several months or more. ECT may be available to some palliative care–based clinicians, particularly those practicing in tertiary care centers. Consideration of ECT should always involve consultation with a psychiatrist.

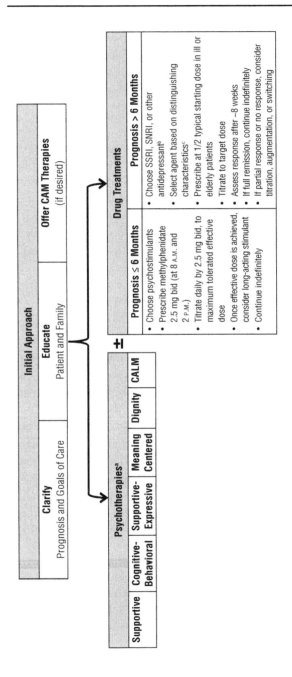

Figure 3–1.   Overview of the management of depression in the palliative care setting.   CALM = Managing Cancer and Living Meaningfully; CAM = complementary and alternative medicine; SNRI = serotonin-norepinephrine reuptake inhibitor; SSRI = selective serotonin reuptake inhibitor. [a]See Chapter 9, "Psychotherapy." [b]See Table 3–3 ("Drug treatments for major depression in palliative care"). [c]See Table 3–4 ("Factors to consider in choosing an antidepressant in the palliative care setting").

apeutic modalities tested specifically in seriously ill patients, the following have shown particular promise, although data are generally of low to moderate quality and results have been mixed: cognitive-behavioral therapies (Akechi et al. 2008), supportive-expressive group therapy (Kissane et al. 2007), Dignity Therapy (Chochinov et al. 2011; Julião et al. 2014), Meaning-Centered Psychotherapy (Breitbart et al. 2012), and a brief semistructured intervention called Managing Cancer and Living Meaningfully (CALM; Lo et al. 2014). Chapter 9, "Psychotherapy," provides a more detailed review of psychotherapy interventions in the palliative care setting, including those aimed specifically at symptoms of depression.

Complementary Therapies

Several alternative therapies can also be considered when attempting to alleviate depression among patients with serious illness, and some patients may prefer these types of interventions. In a 2010 systematic review looking at the impact of complementary and alternative medicine (CAM) treatments on depression, the American Psychiatric Association Task Force on CAM reported promising results for a variety of modalities, including omega-3 fatty acids, St. John's wort, folate, S-adenosyl-L-methionine (SAMe), acupuncture, light therapy, exercise, and mindfulness psychotherapies (Freeman et al. 2010). Regarding CAM treatments in palliative care populations, some data support the use of music therapy (Hilliard 2005), mindfulness meditation (Shennan et al. 2011), and aromatherapy and massage (Ernst 2009; Fellowes et al. 2008). Although the data supporting the effectiveness of these interventions are generally of low quality, and results are mixed, the interventions entail few harms other than potentially delaying the use of proven therapies such as psychotherapy or medication (Freeman et al. 2010). In addition, caution should be exercised with the use of supplements and "nutraceuticals" with regard to potential drug-drug interactions.

Pharmacotherapy

In general, the drug treatments for depression that are typically used in physically healthy patients are also recommended in palliative care patients, but other agents can play a role in this setting as well. A large meta-analysis and systematic review provided evidence that antidepressant medication therapy in palliative care patients is efficacious, with superiority over placebo achieved by 4–5 weeks and increasing in magnitude with time (Rayner et al. 2011). Of note, for patients with symptoms that do not fit the pattern of a discrete depressive disorder, the role of drug treatments is less clear (and nonpharmacological interventions should be prioritized). However, most (but not all) pharmacological interventions for depression are relatively well tolerated, with few serious side effects and few drug interactions. In the palliative care setting, where there is uncertain effectiveness, diagnostic uncertainty, and low expected harm, many experts in psychiatric palliative care encourage a low threshold to consider carefully supervised, time-limited medication trials— with specialist consultation if these initial strategies are ineffective.

Perhaps most important from the standpoint of medication management of depression in the palliative care setting, drug selection is strongly influenced by consideration of the patient's prognosis. Figure 3–1 illustrates this key decision point: for patients with a prognosis of 6 months or less, psychostimulants are frequently first-line treatments because their time to effect can be much more rapid than standard antidepressants, which are more commonly used with patients with a prognosis of greater than 6 months.

Standard Antidepressants

The antidepressant medications commonly used in palliative care settings are presented in Table 3–3. Among the standard antidepressant drugs, the selective serotonin reuptake inhibitors (SSRIs), such as sertraline and escitalopram, are perhaps the most familiar and widely used. Relative to the tricyclic antidepressants,[5] which used to be considered first-line agents, SSRIs tend to have fewer serious or troublesome adverse effects. The SSRIs commonly cause transient gastrointestinal upset, headache, and dry mouth, and most can cause significant sexual side effects. In addition, recent evidence indicates that some of

---

[5]Tricyclic antidepressants (TCAs) are rarely used for the management of depression in palliative care, due in particular to their anticholinergic effects and the risks of delirium in medically ill patients. However, in patients who do not respond to first-line antidepressants or who have had success in the past with TCAs, these may warrant consideration. TCAs also have good evidence of efficacy in reducing neuropathic pain, but even for this indication the serotonin-norepinephrine reuptake inhibitors (SNRIs) are often preferred due to their favorable side-effect profile.

these drugs (notably, citalopram) carry a dose-dependent risk of QTc interval prolongation. Relative to the SSRIs, the serotonin-norepinephrine reuptake inhibitors (SNRIs), such as venlafaxine and duloxetine, have similar efficacy in treating major depressive disorder; may be more effective in certain anxiety disorders; and have strong data for efficacy in reducing neuropathic pain. SNRIs share a similar side-effect profile with the SSRIs. Finally, several other types of antidepressants with unique mechanisms of action—notably, bupropion and mirtazapine—are also considered first-line antidepressants. Bupropion has mild stimulant properties and is frequently used in patients with significant fatigue or anergia, whereas mirtazapine, at the lower end of its dose range, can improve anorexia and insomnia. Notably, because the standard antidepressants are essentially indistinguishable on the basis of efficacy in alleviating depression, the clinician's familiarity with other unique features, as shown in Table 3–4, will help to guide drug selection. In particular, careful attention should be given to potential drug-drug interactions in view of the high rates of polypharmacy among patients with serious medical illness.

Psychostimulants

Standard antidepressant therapies frequently fall short near the end of life, because the time course to effectiveness can be protracted. Although some patients will experience improvement early in the course of therapy, those who fail to respond quickly need to remain on the drug for roughly 8 weeks at the maximum tolerable dose before response can be adequately gauged (Gelenberg et al. 2010). Multiple drug trials are often necessary to achieve remission. By contrast, psychostimulants have been shown to produce rapid antidepressant effects, and a therapeutic trial can often be completed in a small number of days. For this reason, in situations where the expected prognosis is short, psychostimulants are reasonable first-line agents for treating depression, although systematic reviews of the data have reported mixed results (Candy et al. 2008; Hardy 2009). In one small randomized placebo-controlled trial, methylphenidate was associated with dose-dependent reductions in fatigue, as well as significant, but less robust, improvements in depressive symptoms relative to placebo (Kerr et al. 2012). Typically, stimulant therapy is initiated at a low dose and titrated daily until either the clinical target is reached or unwanted side effects emerge (e.g., anxiety, restlessness, insomnia). Initiating therapy with both a stimulant and a standard antidepressant is not advised,

Table 3–3.   Drug treatments for major depression in palliative care

Drug by class	Suggested dosing, titration	Notes
SSRIs		Less sedation and dry mouth than TCAs Often have sexual side effects Adequate trial requires ~6–8 weeks at therapeutic dose
Citalopram	20 mg/day PO Increase by 10–20 mg/day q 1–2 weeks; max ~40 mg/day PO	Well tolerated Few drug–drug interactions Taper to discontinue, when possible Risk of QTc prolongation at doses >40 mg/day Available routes: PO (tabs, liq)
Escitalopram	10 mg/day PO Increase by 5–10 mg/day q 1–2 weeks; max ~20 mg/day PO	Well tolerated Few drug–drug interactions Taper to discontinue, when possible Available routes: PO (tabs, liq)
Sertraline	50 mg/day PO Increase by 50 mg/day q 1–2 weeks; max ~200 mg/day PO	Well tolerated Few drug–drug interactions Taper to discontinue, when possible Available routes: PO (tabs, liq)

Table 3–3.   Drug treatments for major depression in palliative care *(continued)*

Drug by class	Suggested dosing, titration	Notes
SSRIs *(continued)*		
Fluoxetine	20 mg/day PO Increase by 10–20 mg/day q 1–2 weeks; max ~40 mg/day PO	Many drug-drug interactions Wide dose range: 5–80 mg/day Do not need to taper to discontinue (very long half-life) May be activating in some patients Available routes: PO (tabs, caps, liq)
Paroxetine	20 mg/day PO Increase by 10–20 mg/day q 1–2 weeks; max ~40 mg/day PO	Many drug-drug interactions Significant discontinuation syndrome (very short half-life); taper to discontinue; use caution when oral route is unreliable Available routes: PO (tabs, liq)

Table 3–3.   Drug treatments for major depression in palliative care *(continued)*

Drug by class	Suggested dosing, titration	Notes
SNRIs		Effective adjuncts for neuropathic pain Sometimes have mild stimulant effect Often have sexual side effects Adequate trial requires ~6–8 weeks at therapeutic dose
Venlafaxine	75 mg/day PO (extended release) Increase by 75 mg/day q 1 week; max ~225 mg/day PO	Many common adverse effects (e.g., insomnia, headache, hypertension) Effective in neuropathic pain (higher doses) Significant discontinuation syndrome (very short half-life); taper to discontinue; use caution when oral route is unreliable Extended-release formulation permits daily dosing Available routes: PO (tabs, caps)
Desvenlafaxine	50 mg/day PO	High incidence of gastrointestinal side effects, insomnia, anxiety Major active metabolite of venlafaxine; presumably shares efficacy for depression, anxiety, and neuropathic pain Available routes: PO (tabs)

Table 3–3. Drug treatments for major depression in palliative care (*continued*)

Drug by class	Suggested dosing, titration	Notes
SNRIs (*continued*)		
Duloxetine	30 mg/day PO Increase by 30 mg/day q 1 week; max ~120 mg/day PO	Effective in neuropathic pain Doses >120 mg/day rarely more effective Significant discontinuation syndrome; taper to discontinue; use caution when oral route is unreliable Available routes: PO (caps)
Miscellaneous antidepressants		Effective as single agents; also used to augment effectiveness of SSRI or SNRI
Bupropion	SR formulation: 150 mg PO qam Increase to 150 mg PO bid after ~1 week; max ~200 mg PO bid XL formulation: 150 mg PO qam Increase to 300 mg PO qam after ~1 week; max ~450 mg PO qam	Weak norepinephrine and dopamine reuptake inhibitor Contraindicated with seizures or eating disorders Mild stimulant effect: useful in patients with low energy, but may cause insomnia (twice-daily dosing should be scheduled at 8 A.M. and 2 P.M.) May improve concentration May augment antidepressant effect and reduce sexual side effect of SSRIs Multiple formulations available (IR, SR, XL); XL formulation permits once-daily dosing Available routes: PO (tabs, caps)

Table 3–3.   Drug treatments for major depression in palliative care *(continued)*

Drug by class	Suggested dosing, titration	Notes
Miscellaneous antidepressants *(continued)*		
Mirtazapine	15 mg PO qhs Increase by 15 mg q 1–2 weeks; max ~45 mg PO qhs	Exact mechanism of action unknown (increases central serotonergic and noradrenergic activity) At the lower end of the dose range, causes sedation and stimulates appetite; useful in patients with insomnia and anorexia Causes orthostatic hypotension Available routes: PO (tabs, ODT)
Psychostimulant		Rapid effect, short prognoses
Methylphenidate	2.5 mg PO bid (at 8 A.M. and 2 P.M.) Titrate daily by 2.5 mg bid, to maximum tolerated effective dose	Rapid antidepressant effect Consider first line when prognosis is ≤6 months May cause or worsen anxiety May cause or worsen insomnia Usual effective dose ≤20 mg bid (doses >30 mg/day usually not necessary) Available routes: PO (tabs, caps, liq)

Table 3–3. Drug treatments for major depression in palliative care *(continued)*

Drug by class	Suggested dosing, titration	Notes
Experimental "antidepressant"		
Ketamine	Not recommended	Rapid effect, limited evidence to support clinical use
		Moderate-strength data in healthy populations using intravenous route
		Limited, low-quality data in palliative care or hospice setting; a retrospective chart review and single open-label trial of daily oral administration suggest reductions in depression and anxiety (see text)
		Should be reserved for experimental use until better data are available

Note. Dosing guidelines reflect a general initial strategy based on the clinical experience of the authors and current drug references (Micromedex DRUGDEX 2014). Local experts and other resources should be consulted for specific concerns (e.g., dosing strategies in incomplete responders, or dose adjustments in hepatic/renal insufficiency). All first-line antidepressants in this table (SSRIs, SNRIs, bupropion, mirtazapine) have a U.S. Food and Drug Administration indication for major depressive disorder. For other drugs on this table, treatment of major depression is off-label. bid=twice daily; caps=capsules; IR=immediate release; liq=liquid; max=maximum; ODT=orally disintegrating tablet; PO=per oral; q=every; qam=every morning; qhs=at bedtime; SNRI=serotonin-norepinephrine reuptake inhibitor; SR=sustained release; SSRI=selective serotonin reuptake inhibitor; tabs=tablets; TCA=tricyclic antidepressant; XL=extended release.

Source. Modified from Fairman N, Hirst JM, Irwin SA: "Depression and Anxiety: Assessment and Management in Hospitalized Patients With Serious Illness," in *Hospital-Based Palliative Medicine: A Practical, Evidence-Based Approach.* Edited by Pantilat SZ, Anderson W, Gonzales M, et al. Hoboken, NJ, Wiley, 2015, pp. 71–91. Used with permission.

Table 3–4.   Factors to consider in choosing an antidepressant in the palliative care setting

Factor	Consideration
Prognosis	If the patient's prognosis is ≤6 months, consider psychostimulants as first-line therapy.
Neuropathic pain	If the patient is experiencing neuropathic pain, consider a serotonin-norepinephrine reuptake inhibitor.
Personal history	If the patient has previously experienced response or remission with an antidepressant, consider using the same agent.
Family history	If a family member (in particular, a first-degree relative) has had a favorable response with a particular agent, consider using the same agent.
Common side effects	When possible, choose agents with a side-effect profile that aligns with the patient's symptoms or goals of care. • Example: In patients with anorexia and insomnia, consider mirtazapine. • Example: In patients with anergia or fatigue, consider bupropion.
Presence of anxiety	In a patient with a high level of anxiety, avoid anxiogenic agents, such as fluoxetine, bupropion, or venlafaxine. Also, initiate treatment at a lower dose and titrate more slowly.
Presence of neuropathy	Consider serotonin-norepinephrine reuptake inhibitors or tricyclic antidepressants (see Chapter 10, "Pain Management and Psychopharmacology").
Discontinuation syndromes	If loss of the oral route is anticipated, avoid agents with significant discontinuation syndromes (e.g., paroxetine, venlafaxine); taper to discontinue if possible.

Table 3–4. Factors to consider in choosing an antidepressant in the palliative care setting *(continued)*

Factor	Consideration
Drug-drug interactions	Most first-line antidepressants are CYP substrates, and many also exhibit CYP inhibition. Many have P-glycoprotein activity, although these effects tend to be less well characterized (Sandson et al. 2005). Check drug-drug interactions with a pharmacist or online resource.

Note.   CYP = cytochrome P450; P-glycoprotein = permeability glycoprotein.

Source.   Modified from Fairman N, Hirst JM, Irwin SA: "Depression and Anxiety: Assessment and Management in Hospitalized Patients With Serious Illness," in *Hospital-Based Palliative Medicine: A Practical, Evidence-Based Approach.* Edited by Pantilat SZ, Anderson W, Gonzales M, et al. Hoboken, NJ, Wiley, 2015, pp. 71–91. Used with permission.

due to problems that arise from polypharmacy (e.g., inability to accurately attribute adverse and beneficial effects). In patients with existing anxiety or with cardiac tachyarrhythmias, alternative agents should be considered, and if stimulant trials are pursued, patients should be monitored closely for adverse effects.

Future Agents

Several agents have recently shown promise in the rapid treatment of depression. Of these, ketamine currently has the strongest evidence: in a series of well-designed randomized trials, intravenous administration of subanesthetic doses of ketamine in medically healthy subjects with depression consistently produced rapid antidepressant effects (Aan Het Rot et al. 2012). Building on this data, a retrospective chart review (Iglewicz et al. 2015) and an open-label pilot study (Irwin et al. 2013) have suggested a potential role for daily oral ketamine in the treatment of depression in hospice patients. Despite these promising results, further investigation will be necessary to firmly establish whether or not ketamine and other novel treatments for depression have roles in palliative care.

Conclusions and Key Points

- Symptoms of depression are common in palliative care settings, and they can range from normal experiences of sadness to clinically significant conditions such as major depression.

- If not identified and effectively addressed, these symptoms can seriously impair quality of life, can increase morbidity and mortality, and may amplify distress in family, caregivers, and clinicians.

- Even in seriously ill patients, including near the very end of life, major depression is frequently treatable.

- Both pharmacological and nonpharmacological interventions are available and effective in the treatment of depression.

- Understanding patients' functional status and prognosis, as well as their broad goals of care, will help to guide interventions when depression is suspected.

- Drug selection in the treatment of major depression in palliative care settings hinges principally on prognosis, and psychostimulants can be an appropriate first-line therapy when the prognosis is short.

References

Aan Het Rot M, Zarate CA Jr, Charney DS, et al: Ketamine for depression: where do we go from here? Biol Psychiatry 72(7):537–547, 2012 22705040

Akechi T, Okuyama T, Onishi J, et al: Psychotherapy for depression among incurable cancer patients. Cochrane Database Syst Rev (2):CD005537, 2008 18425922

American Psychiatric Association: Diagnostic and Statistical Manual of Mental Disorders, 5th Edition. Arlington, VA, American Psychiatric Association, 2013

Block SD: Perspectives on care at the close of life. Psychological considerations, growth, and transcendence at the end of life: the art of the possible. JAMA 285(22):2898–2905, 2001 11401612

Block SD; ACP-ASIM End-of-Life Care Consensus Panel. American College of Physicians—American Society of Internal Medicine: Assessing and managing depression in the terminally ill patient. Ann Intern Med 132(3):209–218, 2000 10651602

Breitbart W, Rosenfeld B, Pessin H, et al: Depression, hopelessness, and desire for hastened death in terminally ill patients with cancer. JAMA 284(22):2907–2911, 2000 11147988

Breitbart W, Poppito S, Rosenfeld B, et al: Pilot randomized controlled trial of individual meaning-centered psychotherapy for patients with advanced cancer. J Clin Oncol 30(12):1304–1309, 2012 22370330

Candy M, Jones L, Williams R, et al: Psychostimulants for depression. Cochrane Database Syst Rev (2):CD006722, 2008 18425966

Chochinov HM, Wilson KG, Enns M, et al: Desire for death in the terminally ill. Am J Psychiatry 152(8):1185–1191, 1995 7625468

Chochinov HM, Wilson KG, Enns M, et al: "Are you depressed?" Screening for depression in the terminally ill. Am J Psychiatry 154(5):674–676, 1997 9137124

Chochinov HM, Tataryn D, Clinch JJ, et al: Will to live in the terminally ill. Lancet 354(9181):816–819, 1999 10485723

Chochinov HM, Kristjanson LJ, Breitbart W, et al: Effect of dignity therapy on distress and end-of-life experience in terminally ill patients: a randomised controlled trial. Lancet Oncol 12(8):753–762, 2011 21741309

Ernst E: Massage therapy for cancer palliation and supportive care: a systematic review of randomised clinical trials. Support Care Cancer 17(4):333–337, 2009 19148685

Fairman N, Hirst JM, Irwin SA: Depression and anxiety: assessment and management in hospitalized patients with serious illness, in Hospital-Based Palliative Medicine: A Practical, Evidence-Based Approach. Edited by Pantilat SZ, Anderson W, Gonzales M, et al. Hoboken, NJ, Wiley, 2015, pp 71–91

Fellowes D, Barnes K, Wilkinson SS: Aromatherapy and massage for symptom relief in patients with cancer. Cochrane Database Syst Rev (4):CD002287, 2008 18843631

Freeman MP, Fava M, Lake J, et al: Complementary and alternative medicine in major depressive disorder: the American Psychiatric Association Task Force report. J Clin Psychiatry 71(6):669–681, 2010 20573326

Gelenberg AJ, Freeman MP, Markowitz JC, et al: Practice Guideline for the Treatment of Patients With Major Depressive Disorder, 3rd Edition. Arlington, VA, American Psychiatric Association, 2010

Giese-Davis J, Collie K, Rancourt KM, et al: Decrease in depression symptoms is associated with longer survival in patients with metastatic breast cancer: a secondary analysis. J Clin Oncol 29(4):413–420, 2011 21149651

Hardy SE: Methylphenidate for the treatment of depressive symptoms, including fatigue and apathy, in medically ill older adults and terminally ill adults. Am J Geriatr Pharmacother 7(1):34–59, 2009 19281939

Hilliard RE: Music therapy in hospice and palliative care: a review of the empirical data. Evid Based Complement Alternat Med 2(2):173–178, 2005 15937557

Hirdes JP, Freeman S, Smith TF, et al: Predictors of caregiver distress among palliative home care clients in Ontario: evidence based on the interRAI Palliative Care. Palliat Support Care 10(3):155–163, 2012 22436557

Iglewicz A, Morrison K, Nelesen RA, et al: Ketamine for the treatment of depression in patients receiving hospice care: a retrospective medical record review of thirty-one cases. Psychosomatics 56(4):329–337, 2015 25616995

Irwin SA, Fairman N, Montross LP: UNIPAC 2: Alleviating Psychological and Spiritual Pain. UNIPAC Self Study Program, 4th Edition. Edited by Storey CP Jr. Glenview, IL, American Academy of Hospice and Palliative Medicine, 2012

Irwin SA, Iglewicz A, Nelesen RA, et al: Daily oral ketamine for the treatment of depression and anxiety in patients receiving hospice care: a 28-day open-label proof-of-concept trial. J Palliat Med 16(8):958–965, 2013 23805864

Jacobsen JC, Zhang B, Block SD, et al: Distinguishing symptoms of grief and depression in a cohort of advanced cancer patients. Death Stud 34(3):257–273, 2010 20953316

Julião M, Oliveira F, Nunes B, et al: Efficacy of dignity therapy on depression and anxiety in Portuguese terminally ill patients: a phase II randomized controlled trial. J Palliat Med 17(6):688–695, 2014 24735024

Kerr CW, Drake J, Milch RA, et al: Effects of methylphenidate on fatigue and depression: a randomized, double-blind, placebo-controlled trial. J Pain Symptom Manage 43(1):68–77, 2012 22208450

Kissane DW, Clarke DM, Street AF: Demoralization syndrome—a relevant psychiatric diagnosis for palliative care. J Palliat Care 17(1):12–21, 2001 11324179

Kissane DW, Grabsch B, Clarke DM, et al: Supportive-expressive group therapy for women with metastatic breast cancer: survival and psychosocial outcome from a randomized controlled trial. Psychooncology 16(4):277–286, 2007 17385190

Kohout FJ, Berkman LF, Evans DA, Cornoni-Huntley J: Two shorter forms of the CES-D (Center for Epidemiological Studies Depression) depression symptoms index. J Aging Health 5(2):179–193, 1993 10125443

Kroenke K, Spitzer RL, Williams JB: The PHQ-9: validity of a brief depression severity measure. J Gen Intern Med 16(9):606–613, 2001 11556941

Li M, Fitzgerald P, Rodin G: Evidence-based treatment of depression in patients with cancer. J Clin Oncol 30(11):1187–1196, 2012 22412144

Lo C, Hales S, Jung J, et al: Managing Cancer and Living Meaningfully (CALM): phase 2 trial of a brief individual psychotherapy for patients with advanced cancer. Palliat Med 28(3):234–242, 2014 24170718

Micromedex DRUGDEX (Internet database). Ann Arbor, MI, Truven Health Analytics, 2014. Available at: www.micromedexsolutions.com. Subscription required to view.

Mitchell AJ, Meader N, Symonds P: Diagnostic validity of the Hospital Anxiety and Depression Scale (HADS) in cancer and palliative settings: a meta-analysis. J Affect Disord 126(3):335–348, 2010 20207007

Mitchell AJ, Chan M, Bhatti H, et al: Prevalence of depression, anxiety, and adjustment disorder in oncological, haematological, and palliative-care settings: a meta-analysis of 94 interview-based studies. Lancet Oncol 12(2):160–174, 2011 21251875

Rayner L, Price A, Evans A, et al: Antidepressants for the treatment of depression in palliative care: systematic review and meta-analysis. Palliat Med 25(1):36–51, 2011 20935027

Robinson S, Kissane DW, Brooker J, Burney S: A review of the construct of demoralization: history, definitions, and future directions for palliative care. Am J Hosp Palliat Care 33(1):93–101, 2016 25294224

Rodin G, Lo C, Mikulincer M, et al: Pathways to distress: the multiple determinants of depression, hopelessness, and the desire for hastened death in metastatic cancer patients. Soc Sci Med 68(3):562–569, 2009 19059687

Rosenfeld B, Pessin H, Marziliano A, et al: Does desire for hastened death change in terminally ill cancer patients? Soc Sci Med 111:35–40, 2014 24747154

Sandson NB, Armstrong SC, Cozza KL: An overview of psychotropic drug-drug interactions. Psychosomatics 46(5):464–494, 2005 16145193

Satin JR, Linden W, Phillips MJ: Depression as a predictor of disease progression and mortality in cancer patients: a meta-analysis. Cancer 115(22):5349–5361, 2009 19753617

Shennan C, Payne S, Fenlon D: What is the evidence for the use of mindfulness-based interventions in cancer care? A review. Psychooncology 20(7):681–697, 2011 20690112

Spiegel D: Mind matters in cancer survival. JAMA 305(5):502–503, 2011 21285429

Tursi MF, Baes Cv, Camacho FR, et al: Effectiveness of psychoeducation for depression: a systematic review. Aust NZ J Psychiatry 47(11):1019–1031, 2013 23739312

Wasteson E, Brenne E, Higginson IJ, et al; European Palliative Care Research Collaborative (EPCRC): Depression assessment and classification in palliative cancer patients: a systematic literature review. Palliat Med 23(8):739–753, 2009 19825894

Wilson KG, Chochinov HM, Skirko MG, et al: Depression and anxiety disorders in palliative cancer care. J Pain Symptom Manage 33(2):118–129, 2007 17280918

Wilson KG, Lander M, Chochinov HM: Diagnosis and management of depression in palliative care, in Handbook of Psychiatry in Palliative Medicine, 2nd Edition. Edited by Chochinov HM, Breitbart W. New York, Oxford University Press, 2009, pp 39–68

Additional Resources

American Psychiatric Association: DSM-5 Diagnostic Criteria Mobile App. Available for Mac-OS at: https://itunes.apple.com/us/app/dsm-5-diagnostic-criteria/id662938847?mt=8. Available for Android at: https://play.google.com/store/apps/details?id=com.apa.dsm.vandhl=en.

Block SD: Psychological issues in end-of-life care. J Palliat Med 9:751–772, 2006

Education in Palliative and End-of-Life-Care for Oncology (EPEC-Oncology). Module 3h: Depression. Available at: http://www.cancer.gov/cancertopics/cancerlibrary/epeco. Accessed July 20, 2015.

Irwin SA, Fairman N, Montross LP: UNIPAC 2: Alleviating Psychological and Spiritual Pain. UNIPAC Self Study Program, 4th Edition. Edited by Storey CP Jr. Glenview, IL, American Academy of Hospice and Palliative Medicine, 2012. Available at: http://www.aahpm.org/resources/default/unipac-4th-edition.html. Accessed July 20, 2015.

Wilson KG, Lander M, Chochinov HM: Diagnosis and management of depression in palliative care, in Handbook of Psychiatry in Palliative Medicine, 2nd Edition. Edited by Chochinov HM, Breitbart W. New York, Oxford University Press, 2009, pp 39–68

Center to Advance Palliative Care, Fast Facts

Arnold A: Fast Fact #146. Screening for depression in palliative care. Available at: https://www.capc.org/fast-facts/146-screening-depression-palliative-care/. Accessed July 20, 2015.

Jackson V, Block S: Fast Fact #61. Use of psychostimulants in palliative care. Available at: https://www.capc.org/fast-facts/61-use-psycho-stimulants-palliative-care/. Accessed July 20, 2015.

Periyakoil VJ: Fast Fact #43: Is it grief or depression? Available at: https://www.capc.org/fast-facts/43-it-grief-or-depression/. Accessed July 20, 2015.

Warm E, Weissman DE: Fast Fact #7: Depression in advanced cancer. Available at: https://www.capc.org/fast-facts/7-depression-advanced-cancer/. Accessed July 20, 2015.

4

Anxiety

Chapter Overview

Symptoms of anxiety are common among individuals with advanced medical illness. These symptoms range along a continuum from normal, adaptive reactions to stress, to serious and debilitating symptoms that characterize several clinical anxiety disorders. Significant symptoms of anxiety can greatly amplify a patient's suffering. This chapter reviews the approach to identifying and addressing such symptoms in the palliative care setting. The chapter closes with a focus on management strategies for addressing anxiety, including those aimed at long-term treatment of anxiety disorders and those aimed at providing rapid symptom relief.

Symptoms of anxiety are a common source of suffering among patients in palliative care settings. These symptoms can range on a continuum from transient feelings of worry or stress, to the persistent and disabling states of anxiety and associated symptoms that characterize several psychiatric illnesses. Patients in palliative care generally describe anxiety as a feeling of being fearful or overwhelmed, often occurring in connection with physical symptoms (and their potential meaning), practical issues, spiritual crises, or existential concerns as the end of life draws near. Perhaps because of the great stress presumed to accompany an advancing, life-limiting illness, all symptoms of anxiety in this setting are sometimes assumed to be normal or expected experiences, and consequently the more serious forms of anxiety are frequently overlooked or inadequately addressed. Although feeling overwhelmed, worried, or anxious—or even experiencing brief episodes of panic—may be within the range of normal responses to the stress of a serious medical problem, high levels of persistent and disabling anxiety are not an inevitable part of the illness experience in palliative care. Inattention to these symptoms leaves patients and families to suffer needlessly, given that there are many therapeutic strategies that can be effective in ameliorating anxiety, including efforts aimed at practical problem solving and stress reduction, supportive counseling interventions, formal psychotherapy, complementary and alternative therapies, and both short- and long-term drug treatments. Hence, skillful assessment and consideration of evidence-based intervention are warranted whenever patients experience significant anxiety in the palliative care setting.

Epidemiology and Consequences

Epidemiology

Prevalence estimates for anxiety symptoms and anxiety disorders in palliative care vary based on the definitions used and populations studied. Wilson et al. (2007), using a semistructured interview, reported that 14% of patients with advanced cancer met the diagnostic threshold for an anxiety disorder. A large meta-analysis similarly found that anxiety disorders were present in about 9.8% of patients in palliative care settings (Mitchell et al. 2011). Finally, in a large, prospective cohort study of patients with advanced cancer, using a structured clinical interview instrument, Spencer et al. (2010) found that 7.6% of patients met the diagnostic criteria for an anxiety disorder. In the same study, subjects with an anxiety disorder were significantly more likely to be female, to be younger in age, and to have worse performance status, but (perhaps counterintuitively) there was no relationship between an anxiety disorder and the number of medical comorbidities.

Consequences

When unrecognized or ineffectively treated, anxiety can amplify suffering in seriously ill patients and complicate their care. In general adult populations, numerous studies have shown that a high level of psychological distress negatively impacts physical health and quality of life, complicates management of a primary illness, and contributes to significant distress in the patient, loved ones, and clinicians. In palliative care populations specifically, anxiety symptoms are known to reduce quality of life and erode patients' trust in their physicians (Zhang et al. 2012). In a prospective cohort study of adults with advanced cancer, Spencer et al. (2010) found that anxiety disorders seemed to undermine important qualities of the doctor-patient relationship: patients with anxiety were less trustful of their physicians, less comfortable asking health-related questions, less confident that they could comprehend the information their physicians provided, and more likely to believe their physicians would provide futile therapy and would not be able to control their physical symptoms.

Symptoms, Screening, and Differential Diagnosis

Symptoms

Anxiety symptoms may represent a reaction to a psychosocial stressor, a manifestation of a physiological problem, or the hallmark of a serious psychiatric disorder. In palliative care settings, anxiety is frequently described as a feeling of helplessness or fear, often linked to illness-related factors, such as uncontrolled or worsening symptoms, or the prospect of becoming a burden on loved ones. Patients with a short prognosis often worry about death itself. The experience of anxiety can occur in different domains, including emotional, cognitive, behavioral, and physical. Common manifestations of anxiety include the following (Irwin et al. 2012):

- Emotional symptoms: edginess, feelings of impending doom, terror
- Cognitive symptoms: apprehension, dread, obsession, uncertainty, indecision, worry

- Behavioral symptoms: avoidance, compulsions, psychomotor agitation
- Physical symptoms: diaphoresis, diarrhea, nausea, dizziness, tachycardia, tachypnea, dyspnea

In describing their experience, patients often use words such as "concerned," "scared," "worried," or "nervous" to express the psychological experience of anxiety or fear. Attention to these keywords can direct the clinician's attention to the possibility of an anxiety problem (Anderson et al. 2008).

In addition to being psychological responses to a stressor, symptoms of anxiety can also result from physiological derangements related to the underlying medical illness or comorbid conditions. Table 4–1 lists some of the common nonpsychiatric causes of anxiety, which include physical conditions, practical issues, social issues, and existential and spiritual concerns.

Screening

Routine screening for anxiety in palliative care settings can help to identify problematic symptoms and targets for intervention. Several simple screening instruments have been shown to improve the detection of anxiety disorders in general populations. Tools such as the Hospital Anxiety and Depression Scale (Mitchell et al. 2010), the Profile of Mood States (Cella et al. 1987), the four-item Patient Health Questionnaire for Depression and Anxiety (Kroenke et al. 2009), and the Generalized Anxiety Disorder Screener (Löwe et al. 2008) can be helpful, but the performance of these screening tools in palliative care settings has not been thoroughly examined.

Differential Diagnosis

In terms of formal psychiatric conditions, the anxiety-related disorders most commonly encountered in palliative care settings include adjustment disorder, generalized anxiety disorder, panic disorder, and posttraumatic stress disorder (PTSD).[1] Distinguishing features of these conditions are described in detail below and summarized in Table 4–2.

An adjustment disorder results from an identifiable stressor, which produces clinically significant distress (in the form of depression, anxiety, or behavioral disturbances), to a degree that exceeds what would be expected given the severity of the stressor, but not rising to the level of an anxiety disorder. In

Table 4–1. Common nonpsychiatric causes of anxiety in the palliative care setting

Physical conditions

Respiratory failure (dyspnea, hypoxia, increased respiratory effort)

Fatigue, weakness

Uncontrolled pain or other physical symptoms

Insomnia

Hypoglycemia, sepsis, fever, hypertension

Central nervous system malignancy

Drugs (steroids, opioids, withdrawal states, adverse drug reactions such as akathisia)

Delirium

Practical issues

Concerns about finances

Fear of unknown, hospital, or treatment

Uncertainty about future, lack of information, inadequate information

Social issues

Isolation, inadequate support

Concerns about family or caregivers

Disrupted family or peer relationships

Existential and spiritual concerns

Religious doubt, loss of faith

Loss of role

Sense of purposelessness

Hopelessness

---

[1]In the *Diagnostic and Statistical Manual of Mental Disorders,* 5th Edition (American Psychiatric Association 2013), PTSD and adjustment disorder are classified in a new category, Trauma- and Stressor-Related Disorders. Generalized anxiety disorder and panic disorder remain in the category of Anxiety Disorders.

Table 4–1. Common nonpsychiatric causes of anxiety in the palliative care setting *(continued)*

Existential and spiritual concerns *(continued)*

  Fear of mental impairment or loss of cognition or awareness

  Fear of loss of independence

  Fear of dying

  Feelings of guilt or regret

Source.   Modified from Irwin SA, Fairman N, Montross LP: *UNIPAC 2: Alleviating Psychological and Spiritual Pain. UNIPAC Self Study Program,* 4th Edition. Edited by Storey CP Jr. Glenview, IL, American Academy of Hospice and Palliative Medicine, 2012. Used with permission.

an adjustment disorder, by definition, symptoms do not fit the clear pattern of a true anxiety disorder, and—at least in theory—resolution or removal of the stressor should lead to improvement in symptoms (American Psychiatric Association 2013). This distinction is important because, in anxiety disorders, often there is no identifiable stressor or the symptoms persist in the absence of a clear trigger. For some individuals, an adjustment disorder can result from the difficulty associated with adaptation to the diagnosis of a serious illness, realization of its prognosis, difficulties with a treatment regimen, or other stressful circumstances related to the illness.

Worry is the core feature of generalized anxiety disorder, a condition characterized by excessive, persistent, and uncontrollable worry, causing significant functional impairment and occurring over a period of at least 6 months. Patients with generalized anxiety disorder are often described as "worriers" by friends or family members. Associated features can include psychological symptoms, such as apprehension or irritability, and physical (or somatic) symptoms, such as fatigue or muscle tension (American Psychiatric Association 2013).

Recurrent panic attacks are the hallmark of panic disorder, along with anxiety around the possibility of future attacks, efforts to avoid attacks or their consequences, and serious functional impairment. Panic attacks are discrete episodes of intense apprehension, fearfulness, terror, or a feeling of impending doom. Symptoms usually begin abruptly, peak quickly, and last on the order

Table 4–2. Anxiety disorders commonly encountered in the palliative care setting

Condition	Characteristics	General approach to treatment
Adjustment disorder with anxiety	Emotional or behavioral symptoms that develop within 3 months of an identifiable stressor.	Supportive counseling aimed at bolstering coping skills
	Symptoms are disproportionate to the severity or intensity of the stressor.	Problem solving aimed at resolving or removing the stressor
	May occur with features of depression, anxiety, or behavior, or any combination.	Symptom-focused, time-limited drug treatments
	Symptoms do not meet criteria for any particular anxiety disorder.	
Generalized anxiety disorder	A state of excessive and uncontrollable anxiety or worry, lasting at least 6 months and impacting day-to-day activities.	Psychotherapy + drug therapy
	People suffering with generalized anxiety are often described as worriers by their friends and families.	
	Estimated prevalence in advanced cancer = 3%.	

Table 4–2.   Anxiety disorders commonly encountered in the palliative care setting *(continued)*

Condition	Characteristics	General approach to treatment
Panic attack or panic disorder	*Panic attack:* Sudden onset of intense terror, apprehension, fearfulness, or feeling of impending doom, usually accompanied by shortness of breath, palpitations, chest discomfort, a sense of choking, fear of "going crazy" or losing control, often in unexpected situations. Panic attacks are discrete, usually lasting 15–20 minutes. *Panic disorder:* Marked by recurrent panic attacks, accompanied by worry about future attacks, with significant impairment in psychosocial functioning. Estimated prevalence in advanced cancer = 3%.	Psychotherapy (cognitive-behavioral) + drug therapy
Posttraumatic stress disorder	Reexperiencing of a traumatic event, with symptoms of increased arousal, nightmares, intrusive memories, hypervigilance, and avoidance of reminders of the event. Estimated prevalence in advanced cancer = 3.2%.	Psychotherapy (exposure, cognitive-behavioral) + drug therapy

Note.   Descriptions of disorders based on DSM-5 (American Psychiatric Association 2013). Prevalence estimates based on Spencer et al. (2010).

Source.   Modified from Fairman N, Hirst JM, Irwin SA: "Depression and Anxiety: Assessment and Management in Hospitalized Patients With Serious Illness," in *Hospital-Based Palliative Medicine: A Practical, Evidence-Based Approach.* Edited by Pantilat SZ, Anderson W, Gonzales M, et al. Hoboken, NJ, Wiley, 2015, pp. 71–91. Used with permission.

of minutes. Autonomic symptoms such as chest discomfort, shortness of breath, or palpitations are common (American Psychiatric Association 2013).

PTSD occurs after exposure to significant trauma, resulting in reexperiencing phenomena (e.g., nightmares or intrusive memories), hyperarousal, and symptoms of avoidance—all contributing to considerable social, occupational, and interpersonal dysfunction. In palliative care, PTSD is sometimes seen in connection with the experience of receiving a difficult diagnosis or poor prognosis, or from treatment-related events, such as receiving chemotherapy or radiation or undergoing an emergency intubation (Abbey et al. 2015; Kangas et al. 2002; Long et al. 2014).

Management of Anxiety in the Palliative Care Setting

The general approach to addressing anxiety in seriously ill patients should be rooted in basic principles of palliative care: interventions need to be informed by knowledge of prognosis and goals of care, optimal care is provided by a transdisciplinary team, physical symptoms and other dimensions of distress need to be assessed and addressed, nonpharmacological interventions should be optimized, and pharmacological treatments should be provided in the context of time-limited therapeutic trials with clear clinical goals.

As discussed in Chapter 1, "Palliative Care 101," the term *goals of care* refers to the aims of medical therapy in relation to the patient's values and preferences. Because anxiety can be such a common and distressing experience in seriously ill patients, when goals of care are aimed at comfort, significant symptoms often warrant clinical attention and consideration of symptom-focused treatment, even in the absence of a formal psychiatric illness. In such cases, pharmacotherapy often involves off-label drug treatments, further underscoring the need for a careful clarification of goals with the patient and family and the potential benefit of psychiatric consultation.

For patients with anxiety, as for those with depression, a goals clarification may uncover preferences about management that are influenced by stigma or prior experience with mental health treatment, which ought to be sensitively explored with the patient and family as part of the process of developing a care plan. Fully informed decision making in this setting requires a thorough discussion of the medical situation (including the expected prognosis, likely etiology and classification of anxiety symptoms, and risks and burdens associated with potential interventions), *complemented by* an explication of the patient's goals under the circumstances.

A thorough assessment for anxiety includes 1) a detailed history and physical examination focused on psychosocial stressors and other conditions that could potentially cause or exacerbate anxiety; 2) a review of lifestyle factors, behaviors, and substances that may contribute to anxiety (e.g., sleep habits, smoking, use of alcohol or caffeine); 3) laboratory testing, if consistent with goals, to screen for medical conditions associated with anxiety, including electrolytes, blood cell counts, relevant hormones (e.g., thyroid and adrenal), and toxicology; and 4) collateral information from family, friends, and members of the care team (Irwin et al. 2012).

Management strategies for depression and anxiety overlap substantially; many psychotherapy interventions for depression are also useful in the management of anxiety, and even the standard drug treatments are often effective as long-term therapy for both conditions. In treating anxiety, comprehensive management involves addressing any reversible contributors to anxiety (e.g., practical concerns, medication side effects); managing physical symptoms linked to anxiety, such as shortness of breath (e.g., by using opioids); and implementing a variety of nonpharmacological and drug treatment strategies aimed at either immediate or long-term symptom relief. Figure 4–1 provides an overview of the general approach to managing anxiety symptoms in palliative care settings.

Psychotherapy

Chapter 9, "Psychotherapy," provides a more detailed discussion of psychotherapy interventions in the palliative care setting, including a review of general supportive counseling strategies that can be helpful in beginning to address anxiety. More formal therapy approaches can be helpful for patients and families by providing a forum to explore root causes of anxiety symptoms, such as concerns about medical interventions, physical symptoms, finances, disability, dependency, becoming a burden, spiritual issues, existential questions, disease progression, prognosis, or fears about dying (Irwin et al. 2012).

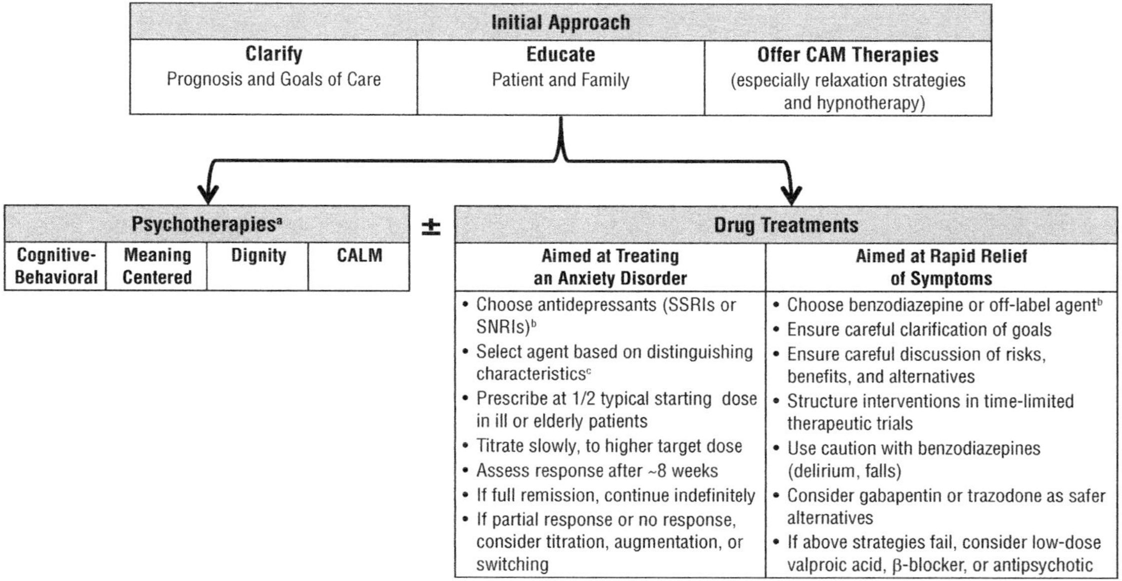
Initial Approach
Clarify
Prognosis and Goals of Care
Educate
Patient and Family
Offer CAM Therapies
(especially relaxation strategies and hypnotherapy)
Psychotherapies[a]
Cognitive-Behavioral
Meaning Centered
Dignity
CALM
±
Drug Treatments
Aimed at Treating an Anxiety Disorder
• Choose antidepressants (SSRIs or SNRIs)[b]
• Select agent based on distinguishing characteristics[c]
• Prescribe at 1/2 typical starting dose in ill or elderly patients
• Titrate slowly, to higher target dose
• Assess response after ~8 weeks
• If full remission, continue indefinitely
• If partial response or no response, consider titration, augmentation, or switching
Aimed at Rapid Relief of Symptoms
• Choose benzodiazepine or off-label agent[b]
• Ensure careful clarification of goals
• Ensure careful discussion of risks, benefits, and alternatives
• Structure interventions in time-limited therapeutic trials
• Use caution with benzodiazepines (delirium, falls)
• Consider gabapentin or trazodone as safer alternatives
• If above strategies fail, consider low-dose valproic acid, β-blocker, or antipsychotic

Figure 4–1. Overview of the management of anxiety symptoms in the palliative care setting. CALM = Managing Cancer and Living Meaningfully; CAM = complementary and alternative medicine; SNRI = serotonin-norepinephrine reuptake inhibitor; SSRI = selective serotonin reuptake inhibitor. [a]See Chapter 9, "Psychotherapy." [b]See Table 4–3 ("Drug treatments for anxiety in palliative care"). [c]See Table 3–4 ("Factors to consider in choosing an antidepressant in the palliative care setting") in Chapter 3, "Depression."

Several psychotherapy modalities aimed at patients with serious medical illness have shown promise for improving symptoms of anxiety, including cognitive-behavioral therapies (Greer et al. 2012), Dignity Therapy (Julião et al. 2014), and group-based Meaning-Centered Psychotherapy (Breitbart et al. 2010). Concreteness training, a brief intervention targeting cognitions centered on worry and rumination, has been shown to reduce anxiety symptoms in a small randomized controlled trial in the hospice setting (Galfin et al. 2012).

Complementary Therapies

As in the management of depression (see Chapter 3, "Depression"), complementary and alternative medicine (CAM) therapies can be considered when attempting to ameliorate anxiety symptoms in patients with serious illness, and some patients may prefer these types of interventions. Regarding CAM treatments for anxiety in palliative care populations, some data support the use of music therapy (Hilliard 2005), mindfulness meditation (Shennan et al. 2011), aromatherapy and massage (Ernst 2009; Fellowes et al. 2004), and hypnotherapy. With respect to hypnotherapy, a small open-label trial in an inpatient hospice unit reported that a brief hypnotherapy intervention was associated with prompt and sustained reductions in symptoms of anxiety (Plaskota et al. 2012). Although the data supporting the effectiveness of CAM interventions are generally of low quality, and results are mixed, the interventions entail few harms apart from the potential delay in implementing proven therapies such as psychotherapy or medication (Freeman et al. 2010).

Pharmacotherapy

A substantial body of high-quality evidence supports combined treatment using medication and psychotherapy for otherwise healthy patients with anxiety disorders. In individuals with symptoms of anxiety that do not fit the clear diagnostic pattern of a psychiatric illness, however, the role of drug treatments is less clear. A Cochrane review found insufficient evidence to guide pharmacological treatment of anxiety in adult palliative care populations (Candy et al. 2012), underscoring the importance of optimizing nonpharmacological interventions and ensuring that medication strategies, when used, are aligned with the patient's goals and are structured in time-limited therapeutic trials.

Fortunately, many (but not all) drug therapies for anxiety are relatively well tolerated, and they have few serious potential side effects and few drug interactions. In this setting, where there is uncertain effectiveness but low likelihood of harm, many experts in psychiatric palliative care encourage a low threshold to consider carefully supervised, time-limited therapeutic trials of medication—with consideration of a specialist referral if initial interventions are ineffective.

Drug treatment strategies for anxiety in palliative care can be conceptualized in two broad categories:

1. Long-term strategies aimed at treatment of anxiety disorders—typically involving the use of antidepressant medications
2. Short-term strategies aimed at rapid symptom relief—typically involving either benzodiazepines or off-label use of other agents with anxiolytic properties

Table 4–3 provides details about drugs commonly used for the management of anxiety in palliative care.

Antidepressants

For long-term management of anxiety disorders, antidepressants are the mainstay of medication treatment. Their use is supported by abundant evidence, and the strategies and agents typically used in healthy patients can also be recommended in palliative care settings. The most commonly used agents include selective serotonin reuptake inhibitors (SSRIs), such as sertraline and escitalopram, and serotonin-norepinephrine reuptake inhibitors (SNRIs), such as venlafaxine and duloxetine. As noted in Chapter 10, "Pain Management and Psychopharmacology," strong evidence supports a role for SNRIs as adjuvant analgesic agents in the management of neuropathic pain, a feature that distinguishes them from SSRIs. In fact, because some data suggest that SNRIs produce a relatively swift and robust antineuropathic effect (relative to a longer time to effect in treating depression or anxiety), in patients with a prognosis of 6 months or less who experience both anxiety and neuropathy, it is reasonable to initiate treatment with an SNRI and to simultaneously consider drug therapy aimed at rapid symptom relief of anxiety.

Table 4–3. Drug treatments for anxiety in palliative care

Drug by class	Suggested dosing, titration	Notes
Long-term strategies aimed at treatment of anxiety disorders		
SSRIs		Often have sexual side effects Adequate trial requires ~6–8 weeks at therapeutic dose
Citalopram	10 mg/day PO Increase by 10 mg/day q 2 weeks; max ~40 mg/day PO	Well tolerated; few drug-drug interactions Taper to discontinue, when possible Risk of QTc prolongation at doses >40 mg/day Available routes: PO (tabs, liq)
Escitalopram	5 mg/day PO Increase by 5–10 mg/day q 2 weeks; max ~20 mg/day PO	Well-tolerated; few drug-drug interactions Taper to discontinue, when possible Available routes: PO (tabs, liq)
Sertraline	25 mg/day PO Increase by 25–50 mg/day q 2 weeks; max ~200 mg/day PO	Well-tolerated; few drug-drug interactions Taper to discontinue, when possible Available routes: PO (tabs, liq)
Fluoxetine	10 mg/day PO Increase by 10 mg/day q 2 weeks; max ~60 mg/day PO	Many drug-drug interactions Wide dose range: 5–80 mg/day Do not need to taper to discontinue (very long half-life) May be activating in some patients Available routes: PO (tabs, caps, liq)

Table 4–3. Drug treatments for anxiety in palliative care *(continued)*

Drug by class	Suggested dosing, titration	Notes
Long-term strategies aimed at treatment of anxiety disorders (continued)		
SSRIs *(continued)*		
Paroxetine	10 mg/day PO Increase by 10 mg/day q 2 weeks; max ~60 mg/day PO	Many drug-drug interactions Significant discontinuation syndrome (very short half-life); taper to discontinue; use caution when oral route is unreliable Available routes: PO (tabs, liq)
SNRIs		Effective adjuncts for neuropathic pain Sometimes have a mild stimulant effect Often have sexual side effects Adequate trial requires ~ 6–8 weeks at therapeutic dose
Venlafaxine	37.5 mg/day PO (extended release) Increase by 37.5 mg/day q 2 weeks; max ~225 mg/day PO	Many common adverse effects (e.g., insomnia, headache, hypertension) Effective in neuropathic pain (higher doses) Significant discontinuation syndrome (very short half-life); taper to discontinue; use caution when oral route is unreliable Extended-release formulation permits daily dosing Available routes: PO (tabs, caps)

Table 4–3.   Drug treatments for anxiety in palliative care (continued)

Drug by class	Suggested dosing, titration	Notes
Long-term strategies aimed at treatment of anxiety disorders (continued)		
SNRIs (continued)		
Desvenlafaxine	50 mg/day PO	High incidence of gastrointestinal side effects, insomnia, anxiety Active metabolite of venlafaxine; presumably efficacious in depression, anxiety, and neuropathic pain Available routes: PO (tabs)
Duloxetine	30 mg/day PO Increase by 30 mg/day q 2 weeks; max ~120 mg/day PO	Effective in neuropathic pain Significant discontinuation syndrome; taper to discontinue; use caution when oral route is unreliable Available routes: PO (caps)
Miscellaneous antidepressants		
Bupropion		Minimal data support the efficacy of bupropion in anxiety disorders, and it cannot be recommended for this purpose.
Mirtazapine		Minimal data suggest that mirtazapine may affect anxiety symptoms, but strength of data strongly favors other agents. It does not have FDA approval for the treatment of any anxiety disorder.

Table 4–3.   Drug treatments for anxiety in palliative care *(continued)*

Drug by class	Suggested dosing, titration	Notes
Short-term strategies aimed at rapid relief of symptoms		
Benzodiazepines		Effective anxiolytics, but use with caution in palliative care setting Cause sedation, confusion/delirium, falls, disinhibition Avoid agents with short half-life (e.g., alprazolam)
Lorazepam	0.25–1 mg PO q (60 min prn anxiety Then use "titration strategy" to establish scheduled and prn doses[a]	Wide dose range; adjust to desired effect or side effect, then consider scheduled dose based on demand Half-life: 12–14 hrs Safer in liver failure than clonazepam Available routes: PO (tabs, liq), SL, SC, IM, IV
Clonazepam	0.125–2 mg PO daily or bid Then titrate to effect/side effect	Wide dose range Half-life: 30–40 hrs (despite this, many patients require divided dosing) Slower onset makes it less ideal for prn use Clonazepam 0.25 mg ≈ lorazepam 1 mg Available routes: PO (tabs, ODT)

Table 4–3. Drug treatments for anxiety in palliative care *(continued)*

Drug by class	Suggested dosing, titration	Notes
Short-term strategies aimed at rapid relief of symptoms *(continued)*		
Other agents with "anxiolytic" properties		
Gabapentin	100 mg PO tid	Wide dose range (not to exceed 3 doses or 600 mg/day) Effective in neuropathic pain Requires dose reduction in renal failure Available routes: PO (tabs, caps, liq)
Trazodone	25–50 mg PO q 60 min prn anxiety Then use "titration strategy" to establish scheduled and prn doses[a]	Antidepressant, potentiates CNS serotonergic activity Off-label treatment of insomnia is most common use Adverse effects: sedation, dry mouth, nausea, priapism (rare) Wide dose range; adjust to desired effect/side effect, then consider scheduled dose based on demand (not to exceed 500 mg/day) Available routes: PO (tabs)
Valproic acid	250 mg PO bid Then titrate to effect/side effect	Antiepileptic and mood stabilizer with unknown mechanism of action (involving increased CNS GABA) Avoid or use with caution in hepatic impairment Available routes: PO (caps, liq), IV

Table 4–3. Drug treatments for anxiety in palliative care *(continued)*

Drug by class	Suggested dosing, titration	Notes
Short-term strategies aimed at rapid relief of symptoms *(continued)*		
Other agents with "anxiolytic" properties *(continued)*		
Propranolol	10 mg PO bid Then titrate to effect/side effect	Often used to ameliorate somatic symptoms linked to hyperarousal Watch for hypotension or bradycardia Available routes: PO (tabs, caps, liq), IV
Antipsychotics	e.g., quetiapine 25 mg PO tid e.g., chlorpromazine 25 mg PO tid	Anxiolysis may result from sedating effect Wide dose range, but dose-dependent side effects common in first-generation agents Low risk of extrapyramidal symptoms with quetiapine and chlorpromazine (due to low dopamine receptor affinity)

Note. Dosing guidelines reflect a general strategy based on current drug references (Micromedex DRUGDEX 2014) and the clinical experience of the authors. Local experts and other resources should be consulted for specific concerns (e.g., dosing strategies in incomplete responders, or dose adjustments in hepatic/renal insufficiency). FDA indications for anxiety disorders vary by drug and by the specific disorder, and in practice the first-line antidepressants included here tend to be used interchangeably, although their use may be off-label. Desvenlafaxine does not have FDA approval for any anxiety disorder, but as the active metabolite of venlafaxine, it is expected to have the same efficacy with respect to depression, anxiety, and neuropathy. Use of other agents on this table is off-label with respect to the treatment of anxiety symptoms.   bid=twice daily; caps=capsules; CNS=central nervous system; FDA=U.S. Food and Drug Administration; GABA=γ-aminobutyric acid; IM=intramuscular; IV=intravenous; liq=liquid; max=maximum; ODT=orally disintegrating tablet; PO=per oral; prn=as needed; q=every; SC=subcutaneous; SL=sublingual; SNRI=serotonin-norepinephrine reuptake inhibitor; SSRI=selective serotonin reuptake inhibitor; tabs=tablets; tid=three times daily.
ᵃSee Table 4–4 in this chapter, and Figure 5–2 in Chapter 5, "Delirium."

Source. Modified from Fairman N, Hirst JM, Irwin SA: "Depression and Anxiety: Assessment and Management in Hospitalized Patients With Serious Illness," in *Hospital-Based Palliative Medicine: A Practical, Evidence-Based Approach.* Edited by Pantilat SZ, Anderson W, Gonzales M, et al. Hoboken, NJ, Wiley, 2015, pp. 71–91. Used with permission.

In general, SSRI and SNRI drugs share common adverse effects, including transient gastrointestinal upset, mild headache, and dry mouth. Also, these agents are known to cause significant sexual side effects—a potential outcome that should not be overlooked in palliative care populations. Some of these drugs, particularly citalopram, may carry a dose-dependent risk of QTc prolongation, increasing the chance of a fatal cardiac tachyarrhythmia. Of note, bupropion and mirtazapine, antidepressant agents with unique mechanisms of action, do not appear to have the same efficacy as SSRIs and SNRIs in the treatment of anxiety conditions; there are inconsistent data to support their use in this role.

In general, when using antidepressants to treat long-term anxiety (as compared with their use in the management of depression), the prescribing strategy involves initiating treatment at a lower-than-usual dose, titrating slowly, and aiming for a higher-than-usual target dose. U.S. Food and Drug Administration indications for specific anxiety disorders vary from one drug to another, and there are very limited head-to-head efficacy data supporting the selection of one agent over another. In practice, most clinicians select agents on the basis of other distinguishing characteristics, as discussed in Chapter 3, "Depression" (see Table 3–4).

Benzodiazepines

Among the medication options for rapid relief of anxiety in otherwise healthy individuals, benzodiazepines are the agents of choice. They can provide quick and dependable anxiolysis, as well as (at higher doses) amnesia, sedation, and antiseizure effects, which can become advantageous in treatment near the end of life. Despite these clear benefits in otherwise healthy individuals, however, caution should be exercised when using benzodiazepines in palliative care populations because of their association with many adverse effects in individuals with complex medical illness, including confusion and delirium, gait instability and falls, and excessive sedation. (Concerns surrounding issues with abuse and dependence are often not as pertinent when prognosis is short.)

Benzodiazepines vary primarily based on onset and duration of action, and rational selection of a particular agent is usually driven by knowledge of these differences. When benzodiazepines are indicated in palliative care populations, lorazepam and clonazepam, which are medium- to long-acting drugs, tend to be the main agents used. Of these two, lorazepam is preferred in

patients with hepatic impairment because this medication relies on conjuga-
tive rather than oxidative metabolism. In addition, lorazepam can be dosed for
as-needed use, and it has a role in the relief of both acute anxiety (i.e., panic)
and nausea. The titration technique used to establish scheduled and as-needed
medication doses in hyperactive delirium, as described in Chapter 5, "Delirium" (see Figure 5–2), can also be used with lorazepam in the management of
anxiety; however, providers should anticipate that tolerance will develop over
time. Table 4–4 provides sample orders of as-needed lorazepam based on this
titration strategy. Short-acting agents, such as alprazolam, tend to be avoided
because their short half-life often results in significant rebound anxiety and
can pose concerns about withdrawal if the oral route is lost.

Whichever agent is chosen, the minimum effective dose should be used.
Discontinuation tends to require a taper, with the pace of the taper determined
by the duration of therapy (reducing the dose by 25% per week is often a safe
initial strategy). Although benzodiazepines have an important role in the management of symptoms during the active phase of dying, adverse events tend to
occur more frequently over the last 6 months of a terminal illness, and benzodiazepines may need to be avoided, cross-titrated to longer-acting agents, or
discontinued; however, they can be introduced again during the final days of
life, as symptoms require.

Other Agents

Reliance on standard drug treatments—antidepressants and benzodiazepines—can be problematic in the palliative care setting. The potential delay in
effectiveness and protracted duration of a therapeutic trial can limit the use-
fulness of antidepressants, whereas adverse events often limit the use of benzodiazepines. As a result, off-label drug treatments can be considered in
attempting to ameliorate anxiety in palliative care settings, particularly when
prognosis is short, suffering is high, or standard treatments have proved ineffective or harmful.

Several agents, from different classes and with different mechanisms, have
been used for short-term, rapid symptom relief from anxiety; their use is based
largely on clinical practice, anecdotal evidence, and knowledge of common
side effects. Gabapentin and trazodone, for example, may have some impact
on symptoms of anxiety (Mavissakalian et al. 1987; Pande et al. 2000), and
they are often used off-label in an as-needed role in palliative care settings.

Table 4–4. Sample orders for as-needed (prn) dosing to address anxiety

Lorazepam	Trazodone
To control:	To control:
• 0.5 mg PO q 60 min prn anxiety	• 50 mg PO q 60 min prn anxiety
• If 3 doses not effective, call physician to reassess dose, diagnosis, or medication choice.	• If 3 doses not effective, call physician to reassess dose, diagnosis, or medication choice.
Once controlled:	Once controlled:
• Schedule the total dose given in the last 24 hours, using divided doses given 2–4 times daily.	• Schedule the total dose used in the last 24 hours in 2–3 divided doses given every 8–12 hours.
• Continue using the prn dose that was previously effective	• Continue using the prn dose that was previously effective.
Caution: Do not exceed 40 mg/day.	*Caution: Do not exceed 500 mg/day.*

Note. PO = per oral; q = every.

Each can provide effective and rapid relief from anxiety symptoms in some patients, and adverse events appear to be minimal. Gabapentin has the added advantage of being effective in neuropathic pain; it also can help improve sleep and has few drug interactions. Trazodone has a wide dose range in the management of anxiety. Common side effects of trazodone can include sedation, dry mouth, and nausea; priapism is a rare but serious complication. Table 4–4 provides sample orders of as-needed lorazepam. Low doses of valproic acid may have a role in the off-label management of anxiety symptoms as well. Buspirone is often tried, but it is not effective as an as-needed agent and seems to benefit only certain patients. β-Blockers may provide some benefit in alleviating the somatic symptoms that accompany hyperarousal. Finally, some sources have advocated a limited role for low-dose antipsychotic drugs to target anxiety on an as-needed basis, particularly for patients in whom delirium may be a concern (Roth and Massie 2009). For example, quetiapine, an antipsychotic with very low dopamine receptor affinity (and, therefore, low risk of symptoms), causes mild sedation at low doses, and some patients report satisfactory anxiolysis with this agent (Buoli et al. 2013). Unfortunately, solid evidence for most of these therapies, beyond clinical experience, is lacking. Hence, careful discussion with patients and families and close monitoring of time-limited goal-oriented trials for improvement or adverse effects should be essential parts of the care plan when addressing symptoms of anxiety.

Conclusions and Key Points

- Symptoms of anxiety are common among patients with serious, advanced illness, and the symptoms range along a continuum from normal, adaptive reactions to stress, to the serious and debilitating symptoms that characterize several clinical anxiety disorders.

- When unrecognized or ineffectively addressed, symptoms of anxiety contribute to poor quality of life, and they can undermine important dimensions of the doctor-patient relationship.

- Nonpharmacological interventions to reduce anxiety include problem-solving interventions, relaxation strategies, complementary and alternative medicine treatments, and a variety of formal psychotherapy approaches.

- Pharmacological interventions to reduce anxiety can be categorized as 1) those aimed at treating anxiety disorders (typically with antidepressants) and 2) those aimed at providing short-term, rapid relief (typically with benzodiazepines or off-label medications).

- Benzodiazepines are effective anxiolytics, but in seriously ill patients they can be associated with significant adverse events.

- Although there is little empirical evidence to guide off-label medication use in addressing anxiety in palliative care, clinical experience supports the use of several agents, such as gabapentin, trazodone, and valproic acid.

References

Abbey G, Thompson SB, Hickish T, et al: A meta-analysis of prevalence rates and moderating factors for cancer-related post-traumatic stress disorder. Psycho-oncology 24(4):371–381, 2015 25146298

American Psychiatric Association: Diagnostic and Statistical Manual of Mental Disorders, 5th Edition. Arlington, VA, American Psychiatric Association, 2013

Anderson WG, Alexander SC, Rodriguez KL, et al: "What concerns me is…" Expression of emotion by advanced cancer patients during outpatient visits. Support Care Cancer 16(7):803–811, 2008 17960430

Breitbart W, Rosenfeld B, Gibson C, et al: Meaning-centered group psychotherapy for patients with advanced cancer: a pilot randomized controlled trial. Psychooncology 19(1):21–28, 2010 19274623

Buoli M, Caldiroli A, Caletti E, et al: New approaches to the pharmacological management of generalized anxiety disorder. Expert Opin Pharmacother 14(2):175–184, 2013 23282069

Candy B, Jackson KC, Jones L, et al: Drug therapy for symptoms associated with anxiety in adult palliative care patients. Cochrane Database Syst Rev 10:CD004596, 2012 23076905

Cella DF, Jacobsen PB, Orav EJ, et al: A brief POMS measure of distress for cancer patients. J Chronic Dis 40(10):939–942, 1987 3611291

Ernst E: Massage therapy for cancer palliation and supportive care: a systematic review of randomised clinical trials. Support Care Cancer 17(4):333–337, 2009 19148685

Fairman N, Hirst JM, Irwin SA: Depression and anxiety: assessment and management in hospitalized patients with serious illness, in Hospital-Based Palliative Medicine: A Practical, Evidence-Based Approach. Edited by Pantilat SZ, Anderson W, Gonzales M, et al. Hoboken, NJ, Wiley, 2015, pp 71–91

Fellowes D, Barnes K, Wilkinson S: Aromatherapy and massage for symptom relief in patients with cancer. Cochrane Database Syst Rev (2):CD002287, 2004 15106172

Freeman MP, Fava M, Lake J, et al: Complementary and alternative medicine in major depressive disorder: the American Psychiatric Association Task Force report. J Clin Psychiatry 71(6):669–681, 2010 20573326

Galfin JM, Watkins ER, Harlow T: A brief guided self-help intervention for psychological distress in palliative care patients: a randomised controlled trial. Palliat Med 26(3):197–205, 2012 21807750

Greer JA, Traeger L, Bemis H, et al: A pilot randomized controlled trial of brief cognitive-behavioral therapy for anxiety in patients with terminal cancer. Oncologist 17(10):1337–1345, 2012 22688670

Hilliard RE: Music therapy in hospice and palliative care: a review of the empirical data. Evid Based Complement Alternat Med 2(2):173–178, 2005 15937557

Irwin SA, Fairman N, Montross LP: UNIPAC 2: Alleviating Psychological and Spiritual Pain. UNIPAC Self Study Program, 4th Edition. Edited by Storey CP Jr. Glenview, IL, American Academy of Hospice and Palliative Medicine, 2012

Julião M, Oliveira F, Nunes B, et al: Efficacy of dignity therapy on depression and anxiety in Portuguese terminally ill patients: a phase II randomized controlled trial. J Palliat Med 17(6):688–695, 2014 24735024

Kangas M, Henry JL, Bryant RA: Posttraumatic stress disorder following cancer. A conceptual and empirical review. Clin Psychol Rev 22(4):499–524, 2002 12094509

Kroenke K, Spitzer RL, Williams JB, Löwe B: An ultra-brief screening scale for anxiety and depression: the PHQ-4. Psychosomatics 50(6):613–621, 2009 19996233

Long AC, Kross EK, Davydow DS, Curtis JR: Posttraumatic stress disorder among survivors of critical illness: creation of a conceptual model addressing identification, prevention, and management. Intensive Care Med 40(6):820–829, 2014 24807082

Löwe B, Decker O, Müller S, et al: Validation and standardization of the Generalized Anxiety Disorder Screener (GAD-7) in the general population. Med Care 46(3): 266–274, 2008 18388841

Mavissakalian M, Perel J, Bowler K, et al: Trazodone in the treatment of panic disorder and agoraphobia with panic attacks. Am J Psychiatry 144(6):785–787, 1987 3296792

Micromedex DRUGDEX (Internet database). Ann Arbor, MI, Truven Health Analytics, 2014. Available at: www.micromedexsolutions.com. Subscription required to view.

Mitchell AJ, Meader N, Symonds P: Diagnostic validity of the Hospital Anxiety and Depression Scale (HADS) in cancer and palliative settings: a meta-analysis. J Affect Disord 126(3):335–348, 2010 20207007

Mitchell AJ, Chan M, Bhatti H, et al: Prevalence of depression, anxiety, and adjustment disorder in oncological, haematological, and palliative-care settings: a meta-analysis of 94 interview-based studies. Lancet Oncol 12(2):160–174, 2011 21251875

Pande AC, Pollack MH, Crockatt J, et al: Placebo-controlled study of gabapentin treatment of panic disorder. J Clin Psychopharmacol 20(4):467–471, 2000 10917408

Plaskota M, Lucas C, Evans R, et al: A hypnotherapy intervention for the treatment of anxiety in patients with cancer receiving palliative care. Int J Palliat Nurs 18(2):69–75, 2012 22399044

Roth AJ, Massie MJ: Anxiety in palliative care, in Handbook of Psychiatry in Palliative Medicine, 2nd Edition. Edited by Chochinov HM, Breitbart W. New York, Oxford University Press, 2009, pp 69–80

Shennan C, Payne S, Fenlon D: What is the evidence for the use of mindfulness-based interventions in cancer care? A review. Psychooncology 20(7):681–697, 2011 20690112

Spencer R, Nilsson M, Wright A, et al: Anxiety disorders in advanced cancer patients: correlates and predictors of end-of-life outcomes. Cancer 116(7):1810–1819, 2010 20187099

Wilson KG, Chochinov HM, Skirko MG, et al: Depression and anxiety disorders in palliative cancer care. J Pain Symptom Manage 33(2):118–129, 2007 17280918

Zhang B, Nilsson ME, Prigerson HG: Factors important to patients' quality of life at the end of life. Arch Intern Med 172(15):1133–1142, 2012 22777380

Additional Resources

American Psychiatric Association: DSM-5 Diagnostic Criteria Mobile App. Available for Mac-OS at: https://itunes.apple.com/us/app/dsm-5-diagnostic-criteria/id662938847?mt=8. Available for Android at: https://play.google.com/store/apps/details?id=com.apa.dsm.vandhl=en.

Block SD: Psychological issues in end-of-life care. J Palliat Med 9:751–772, 2006

Education in Palliative and End-of-Life-Care for Oncology (EPEC-Oncology). Module 3c: Anxiety. Available at: http://www.cancer.gov/cancertopics/cancerlibrary/epeco. Accessed July 20, 2015.

Irwin SA, Fairman N, Montross LP: UNIPAC 2: Alleviating Psychological and Spiritual Pain. UNIPAC Self Study Program, 4th Edition. Edited by Storey CP Jr. Glenview, IL, American Academy of Hospice and Palliative Medicine, 2012. Available at: http://www.aahpm.org/resources/default/unipac-4th-edition.html. Accessed July 20, 2015.

Irwin SA, Montross LP, Chochinov HM: What treatments are effective for anxiety in patients with serious illness? in Evidence-Based Practice of Palliative Medicine. Edited by Goldstein NE, Morrison RS. Philadelphia, PA, Elsevier Saunders, 2012, pp 191–197

Roth AJ, Massie MJ: Anxiety in palliative care, in Handbook of Psychiatry in Palliative Medicine, 2nd Edition. Edited by Chochinov HM, Breitbart W. New York, Oxford University Press, 2009, pp 69–80

Center to Advance Palliative Care, Fast Facts

Cooper K, Stollings S: Fast Fact #211: Guided imagery for anxiety. Available at: https://www.capc.org/fast-facts/211-guided-imagery-anxiety/. Accessed July 20, 2015.

Periyakoil VJ: Fast Fact #145: Panic disorder at the end-of-life. Available at: https://www.capc.org/fast-facts/145-panic-disorder-end-life/. Accessed July 20, 2015.

Stoklosa J, Patterson J, Roseille DA, et al: Fast Fact #186: Anxiety in palliative care—causes and diagnosis. Available at: https://www.capc.org/fast-facts/186-anxiety-palliative-care-causes-and-diagnosis/. Accessed July 20, 2015.

5

Delirium

Chapter Overview

This chapter reviews the assessment and management of delirium in palliative care settings. Delirium is highly prevalent among patients with serious medical illnesses, and it is associated with many adverse consequences for patients, families, and clinicians. A comprehensive assessment includes careful description of observed symptoms, signs, and behaviors, as well as an understanding of the patient's situation, including primary diagnosis, associated comorbidities, functional status, and prognosis. Patient- and family-centered goals of care must be taken into account, because diagnostic and management strategies differ based on goals of care and potential for reversibility. Both pharmacological and nonpharmacological interventions can improve symptoms and relieve distress, even near the end of life.

Along with depression and anxiety, delirium is one of the most common clinical conditions in palliative care settings for which psychiatrists have unique expertise. Although it is caused by an underlying medical or physiological condition, delirium is manifest by psychiatric symptoms—among them, cognitive changes, perceptual disturbances, and behavioral agitation—

that often trigger the involvement of a psychiatrist, in settings where one is available. Among seriously ill patients, delirium is often misdiagnosed or underrecognized, and it is frequently associated with adverse consequences for patients, caregivers, and clinicians. Moreover, the approach to addressing delirium in the palliative care setting, especially near the very end of life, differs in some important respects from delirium management in other settings. For these reasons, the management of delirium in palliative care is often enhanced by the involvement of an experienced psychiatrist, who can assist by providing an accurate diagnosis, investigating potential etiologies, clarifying the potential for reversibility, and helping to frame achievable goals of care given the particular medical context.

Definition, Epidemiology, Etiologies, Subtypes, and Consequences

Definition

Delirium is an acute change in mental status, marked by a disturbance of attention and other cognitive deficits. Symptoms often fluctuate in severity over the course of a day. By definition, delirium results from an underlying physiological disturbance, such as a significant medical disease, metabolic derangements, the effects of a drug, or multiple etiologies (American Psychiatric Association 2013). Although it has many other names—encephalopathy, acute confusional state, intensive care unit (ICU) psychosis, acute brain failure, or syndrome of cerebral insufficiency, to name a few—the term *delirium* is consistent with psychiatric nomenclature, and use of this term helps to ensure consistency in communication, identification, and management (Irwin et al. 2013).

Epidemiology

Delirium is common in palliative care settings, with prevalence estimates varying widely depending on the population and the method of identification (Hosie et al. 2013). In general, as age and severity of illness increase, so too does the prevalence of delirium: a recent systematic review estimated overall occurrence rates of 29%–64% in general medical and geriatric inpatient wards (Inouye et al. 2014b). Older prospective cohort studies reported prevalence figures of 70% among elderly patients in the ICU (McNicoll et al. 2003) and up to 85% among terminally ill cancer patients (Bruera et al. 1992b; Massie et al. 1983). In patients who are actively dying, rates of delirium probably approach 100%. Nonetheless, despite its high prevalence, delirium is still often missed or misdiagnosed (de la Cruz et al. 2015).

Etiologies

Nearly any disturbance of normal physiology can cause delirium, and patients in palliative care settings are at very high risk for developing delirium because they have complex, dynamic medical problems; are often receiving multiple medications; and are subject to other interventions. Metabolic disturbances, organ failure, medications, infection, and brain pathology are among the etiologies most commonly encountered in the palliative care setting (Casarett et al. 2001; Irwin et al. 2013; LeGrand 2012); additional etiologies are listed in Table 5–1. Among the medications that are typical triggers for delirium are opioids, steroids, benzodiazepines, and anticholinergic agents, each of which frequently has an important role in symptom management in palliative care. In addition, disease-directed therapies, such as chemotherapy and radiation, should also be considered as possible etiologies of delirium.

Delirium has been usefully conceptualized as resulting from a combination of *predisposing* factors and *precipitating* factors; the condition arises in vulnerable patients (e.g., older adults with complex underlying disease and baseline cognitive impairments) who are exposed to new conditions (e.g., use of an anticholinergic medication, or the development of an infection), which together result in delirium (Inouye and Charpentier 1996; Inouye et al. 2014b). Given this, and taking into account the level of medical complexity in seriously ill patients, it is unsurprising that most cases of delirium in palliative care are multifactorial in origin. For example, in a cohort of hospitalized adults with advanced cancer, the median number of precipitating factors was three (Lawlor et al. 2000). Similarly, in a series of over 200 consecutive hospice inpatient admissions, at least two etiological factors were identified in 52% of all cases of delirium (Morita et al. 2001).

Table 5–1. Selected etiologies of delirium in palliative care settings

Common, usually reversible

Medication use (e.g., opioids, benzodiazepines, anticholinergic agents, steroids)

Withdrawal (e.g., benzodiazepines, opioids, alcohol)

Infection (e.g., urinary tract infection, pneumonia)

Constipation

Urinary retention

Dehydration

Less common, usually reversible

Metabolic disturbance (hypo- or hypernatremia, hypo- or hyperglycemia, hypercalcemia)

Anemia

Hypoxemia

Less common, usually irreversible

Organ failure (e.g., renal, hepatic, respiratory)

Central nervous system pathology (e.g., tumor/metastasis, leptomeningeal disease, nonconvulsive status epilepticus)

Source. Adapted from Tucker and Nichols 2012 and LeGrand 2012.

Subtypes

Three subtypes of delirium have been described based on the phenomenology of symptoms (Meagher et al. 2008; Ross et al. 1991; Stagno et al. 2004). Patients with the *hyperactive subtype* may exhibit psychomotor agitation, perceptual disturbances, and/or changes in level of consciousness. In patients with the *hypoactive subtype,* these features are absent; these patients often demonstrate a decreased level of arousal and marked psychomotor retardation, and they may appear profoundly withdrawn or even depressed. Evidence indicates that, contrary to results from earlier studies, a substantial portion of patients with hypoactive delirium also experience perceptual disturbances (50.9%) or delusional thoughts (43.3%) (Boettger and Breitbart 2011). Patients often exhibit features of both hyperactive and hypoactive subtypes, in which case the delirium is classified as the *mixed subtype*. The hypoactive subtype is frequently reported as the most prevalent and most often underrecognized (or misidentified as depression) (Hosie et al. 2013). For example, in one study of 228 hospitalized terminally ill cancer patients, the prevalence of delirium was 46.9%, the hypoactive subtype was most common (68.2%), and the detection rate for the hypoactive subtype was significantly lower than the detection rate for hyperactive or mixed states (Fang et al. 2008). Similarly, in a study of patients receiving inpatient specialist palliative care, hypoactive delirium was the most common subtype, with prevalence estimates ranging from 78% to 86% (Spiller and Keen 2006). Peterson et al. (2006) reported a strong, independent association between older age ($\geq$65 years) and the hypoactive subtype among critically ill patients admitted to a medical ICU. Distinguishing among the subtypes of delirium can be important because the effectiveness of symptom-driven treatments may depend on whether the delirium is predominately hyperactive or hypoactive, as discussed later in this chapter (see "Management of Delirium in the Palliative Care Setting").

Consequences

Delirium is associated with many serious adverse clinical, social, and economic consequences. For patients, the subjective experience of delirium is highly distressful: in a series of patients with advanced cancer who recovered from delirium, for example, 74% remembered the experience of being delirious, and 81% of those rated the experience as distressful (Bruera et al. 2009). Similarly, in a large population of hospitalized patients with cancer, delirium was a source of significant distress, and there were no differences in the level of distress between hyperactive and hypoactive subtypes (Breitbart et al. 2002). These and other studies have also consistently shown high levels of distress among family members and caregivers in association with observing a loved one with delirium (Bruera et al. 2009; Cohen et al. 2009; Namba et al. 2007).

Delirium has been shown to be associated with serious adverse clinical outcomes, the most significant of which include chronic deficits in cognition (Davis et al. 2012), functional decline (Inouye et al. 1998), and increased mortality, which has been reported in a range of studies using a variety of different methodologies (Cole et al. 2009; Kiely et al. 2009; Lawlor et al. 2000). In a large study of hospitalized older adults, for example, delirium was associated with a 62% increased risk of mortality during the year following discharge, when compared with matched patients without delirium (Leslie et al. 2005). In a meta-analysis, Witlox et al. (2010) showed that delirium is independently associated with an increased risk of institutionalization, dementia, and death, after controlling for age, sex, comorbid illness, severity of illness, and baseline cognitive impairment. There is evidence as well that the presence of delirium can impair the assessment and management of comorbid conditions, such as depression and pain (Breitbart and Alici 2008; Bruera et al. 1992a).

In terms of economic consequences, delirium is strongly associated with increased health care utilization and costs, largely driven by increased hospital admissions, prolonged hospitalizations, and increased need for higher levels of care. Taken together, the total direct costs attributable to delirium have been estimated to range from $143 billion to $152 billion, based on care required during the 1-year period following discharge after an episode of delirium (Leslie and Inouye 2011).

Prevention

Few studies have examined strategies for primary prevention of delirium in palliative care settings (e.g., home-based hospice or inpatient palliative care units). Nonetheless, considerable data exist to support the effectiveness of nonpharmacological prevention strategies in more generalized populations, and on this basis many advocate for similar prevention efforts in palliative care settings, with perhaps some modifications to account for unique contextual considerations (Bush et al. 2014). Most effective prevention efforts involve multicomponent strategies aimed at the numerous predisposing factors and precipitant triggers which, in combination, so often result in delirium. A widely disseminated approach, the Hospital Elder Life Program (HELP), includes elements aimed at early mobilization, reorientation and cognitive engagement, provision of sensory aids (e.g., eyeglasses, hearing aids), promotion and protection of restful sleep, sparing of exposure to psychoactive medication, and maintenance of adequate hydration (Inouye et al. 1999). HELP and similar multicomponent approaches have been shown in several studies in different populations to be effective in the prevention of delirium in at-risk patients (Inouye et al. 2014b; Reston and Schoelles 2013). Of note, prevention strategies appear to provide the greatest benefit in populations known to be at high risk for delirium (those in which prevalence exceeds 30%) (Hempenius et al. 2011). Nonetheless, a multicomponent trial in a group of patients with cancer near the end of life, in whom the prevalence of delirium was 49.1%, failed to show effectiveness (Gagnon et al. 2012). Regarding medication strategies for prevention, data have been mixed and may be of limited generalizability to palliative care populations. On balance, taking into account the quality of data, consistency of results, and considerations about minimizing potential harms, current data support the use of nonpharmacological multicomponent strategies, but not medication, for the purpose of delirium prevention, as reflected in several current practice guidelines (e.g., O'Mahony et al. 2011).

Approach to Delirium in the Palliative Care Setting: Goals of Care, Reversibility, Assessment, and Screening

In palliative care settings, the workup and management of delirium are anchored by the patient's goals of care and the likelihood that reversal of the delirium will be successful. These two features—attention to goals of care and potential for reversibility—have practical consequences for management and distinguish the approach to delirium in palliative care from that in other settings.

Goals of Care

As discussed in Chapter 1, "Palliative Care 101," the term *goals of care* refers to the broad aims of medical therapy in relation to the patient's values and preferences. Ideally, medical care is aimed at enabling patients to achieve the goals that matter most to them, given the circumstances of their particular medical situation and other constraints. With respect to the management of delirium in palliative care, knowledge of goals is critically important because goals guide choices about workup and intervention. Some patients and families, hoping for restoration of a previous level of quality of life, will pursue time-limited therapeutic trials aimed at reversal of the delirium. For them, simple tests, such as blood draws and urinalysis, are acceptable, especially if the results help to identify a simple therapeutic intervention that may potentially reverse the delirium and thereby reduce distress and improve quality of life. For others, ensuring comfort and dignity may be higher priorities, in which case care may focus instead on avoiding burdensome diagnostic testing, managing distressful symptoms, and providing measures aimed purely at the relief of suffering. Fully informed decision making in this setting requires a thorough discussion of the medical situation (including likely causes of delirium, as well as risks and burdens associated with a workup and subsequent intervention), *complemented by* an explication of the patient's goals under the circumstances.

Reversibility

The approach to delirium in the palliative care setting is also guided by careful consideration of whether or not the delirium is reversible. As described in the previous subsection and reflected in Table 5–2, irreversibility may be a result of the goals of care. When the patient's priority is to ensure symptom relief near the end of life, and diagnostic intervention is contrary to the goals of care, the delirium effectively becomes irreversible. In addition, failure to successfully identify the cause of delirium, or inability to successfully reverse it, can also result in a situation in which the delirium is irreversible. Lastly, delirium is also classified as irreversible when it results from a physiological condition that cannot be reversed—such as end-stage organ failure, central nervous system involvement of a tumor, or imminent death.

Nonetheless, studies have consistently shown that even in the context of a serious or advanced illness, the causes of delirium can frequently be identified and at times reversed. For example, Bruera et al. (1992b) reported 33% reversibility in a series of hospitalized adults with terminal cancer. In a prospective cohort study of hospitalized patients with advanced cancer, 49% of all episodes of delirium were successfully reversed (Lawlor et al. 2000). Leonard et al. (2008) followed a series of consecutive palliative care admissions until death; of those who developed delirium, 27% recovered fully from the delirium prior to death.

Table 5–2.   Irreversible delirium

Delirium may be considered irreversible under the following circumstances:

1. **Incompatibility with goals of care**—A diagnostic workup or time-limited therapeutic trial is contrary to goals of care.

2. **Diagnostic failure**—A diagnostic workup fails to identify a reversible etiology of the delirium.

3. **Therapeutic failure**—A time-limited therapeutic trial is unsuccessful at reversing the delirium (even with assistance from expert consultants).

4. **Irreversibility of underlying etiology**—The underlying physiological process is irreversible (e.g., end-stage organ failure, irreversible central nervous system involvement of a tumor, or imminent death).

Assessment

Suspicion for delirium is often raised by acute or subacute changes in arousal, behavior, or perceptual disturbances, although a myriad of features may be present, as reflected in Table 5–3. Given the significant consequences and high prevalence of delirium in palliative care settings, a low threshold of suspicion is warranted. Once delirium is suspected, a careful clinical assessment, anchored by knowledge of the diagnostic criteria (provided in Table 5–4), is necessary to make the diagnosis. In addition to a thorough history, physical examination, and mental status examination, a comprehensive assessment in the palliative care setting also ought to include the following (Irwin et al. 2013):

1. Careful description of the observed behaviors and other clinical signs, as well as their onset and temporal pattern

2. Collateral information from other clinicians and family, who can often contextualize clinical findings and provide essential information about baseline functioning and rapidity of change

3. A clarification of the patient's clinical situation, including the status of the primary underlying disease and its prognosis, its trajectory, relevant co-morbidities, and functional status

4. A clarification of the patient's goals of care, including input from family

5. An understanding of the degree of distress associated with the delirium (as experienced by the patient, family, and other clinicians)

Table 5–3.   Behaviors, symptoms, and signs of delirium

Feature	Definition
Acute onset	Rapid onset of symptoms over minutes to days, even if it began or occurred in the past.
Altered level of consciousness	Altered levels of awareness and alertness (hypervigilant, alert, lethargic, cloudy, stuporous, comatose).
Behavioral agitation	Unintentional, excessive, and purposeless motor activity.
Confusion	Not oriented to person, place, time, or situation.
Delusion	A fixed, false belief or wrong judgment in which opposing evidence does not change a patient's mind; may be paranoid, grandiose, somatic, or persecutory.
Disinhibition	Inability to control immediate or impulsive responses.
Disorganized thinking	Thoughts are confusing or vague, and do not logically flow.
Fluctuation or waxing/waning	Intensity changes rapidly; symptoms may come and go over the course of the day.
Hallucination	Perception of an object or event that does not exist; may be visual, auditory, olfactory, gustatory, or tactile.
Inattention	Inability to focus and direct thinking.
Irritability	Prone to excessive impatience, annoyance, or anger.
Labile affect	Rapid shifts in emotional expression, often discordant with context of mood.
Psychosis	Loss of contact with reality (often marked by delusions or perceptual disturbances).
Restlessness	See "Behavioral agitation" above.

Source.   Adapted from Irwin et al. 2013.

In the palliative care setting, a skilled diagnostician—frequently, a psychiatrist or palliative care specialist—can often assist by helping to 1) differentiate delirium from other related diagnoses, 2) identify its subtype (hyperactive, hypoactive, or mixed), and 3) categorize it as potentially reversible or irreversible.

Table 5–4.   DSM-5 diagnostic criteria for delirium

A.   A disturbance in attention (i.e., reduced ability to direct, focus, sustain, and shift attention) and awareness (reduced orientation to the environment).

B.   The disturbance develops over a short period of time (usually hours to a few days), represents a change from baseline attention and awareness, and tends to fluctuate in severity during the course of a day.

C.   An additional disturbance in cognition (e.g., memory deficit, disorientation, language, visuospatial ability, or perception).

D.   The disturbances in Criteria A and C are not better explained by another preexisting, established, or evolving neurocognitive disorder and do not occur in the context of a severely reduced level of arousal, such as coma.

E.   There is evidence from the history, physical examination, or laboratory findings that the disturbance is a direct physiological consequence of another medical condition, substance intoxication or withdrawal (i.e., due to a drug of abuse or to a medication), or exposure to a toxin, or is due to multiple etiologies.

Specify whether:

Substance intoxication delirium: This diagnosis should be made instead of substance intoxication when the symptoms in Criteria A and C predominate in the clinical picture and when they are sufficiently severe to warrant clinical attention.

Substance withdrawal delirium: This diagnosis should be made instead of substance withdrawal when the symptoms in Criteria A and C predominate in the clinical picture and when they are sufficiently severe to warrant clinical attention.

Medication-induced delirium: This diagnosis applies when the symptoms in Criteria A and C arise as a side effect of a medication taken as prescribed.

Delirium due to another medical condition: There is evidence from the history, physical examination, or laboratory findings that the disturbance is attributable to the physiological consequences of another medical condition.

Delirium due to multiple etiologies: There is evidence from the history, physical examination, or laboratory findings that the delirium has more than one etiology (e.g., more than one etiological medical condition; another medical condition plus substance intoxication or medication side effect).

Table 5–4.   DSM-5 diagnostic criteria for delirium *(continued)*

Specify if:
Acute: Lasting a few hours or days.
Persistent: Lasting weeks or months.

Specify if:
Hyperactive: The individual has a hyperactive level of psychomotor activity that may be accompanied by mood lability, agitation, and/or refusal to cooperate with medical care.
Hypoactive: The individual has a hypoactive level of psychomotor activity that may be accompanied by sluggishness and lethargy that approaches stupor.
Mixed level of activity: The individual has a normal level of psychomotor activity even though attention and awareness are disturbed. Also includes individuals whose activity level rapidly fluctuates.

Note.   Criteria set above contains only the diagnostic criteria and specifiers; refer to DSM-5 for the full criteria set, including coding and reporting procedures.

Source.   DSM-5 criteria for delirium reprinted from *Diagnostic and Statistical Manual of Mental Disorders,* 5th Edition. Washington, DC, American Psychiatric Association, 2013, pp. 596–598. Used with permission. Copyright © 2013 American Psychiatric Association.

Screening

Multiple instruments have been developed to facilitate screening for delirium, and many of these have been recently reviewed, with specific attention to their use in the palliative care setting (Leonard et al. 2014). Of these, perhaps the most widely used is the Confusion Assessment Method, a nine-item instrument that examines the domains of attention, thought process, and level of consciousness over time (Inouye et al. 1990). In a 2010 systematic review encompassing 11 different instruments, the Confusion Assessment Method was shown to have the strongest data (combining test performance and ease of use) supporting its use as a bedside screening instrument (Wong et al. 2010). It can be easily administered by clinicians without psychiatric training, and it has been shown to have high sensitivity (0.94–1.0) and specificity (0.9–0.95) in general populations (Inouye et al. 1990). Although some validation studies have suggested lower test performance in the palliative care setting, after a brief, focused training for nonconsultant physicians in a specialist palliative care unit, sensitivity was 0.88 (0.62–0.98) and specificity was 1.0 (0.88–1.0) (Ryan et al. 2009).

Management of Delirium in the Palliative Care Setting

Most guidelines for the management of delirium recommend interventions aimed simultaneously at four interrelated goals: 1) providing education and support to the patient and family; 2) ensuring safety for the patient, family, and clinicians; 3) addressing the etiological cause(s) of the delirium; and 4) ameliorating symptoms through nonpharmacological and pharmacological strategies. Figure 5–1 provides an overview of the recommended approach to managing delirium in palliative care settings. Of note, for all patients, efforts aimed at family support, patient safety, and nonpharmacological interventions to ameliorate symptoms are appropriate. In contrast, as noted above, overall goals of care and potential for reversibility will shape clinical decisions about a diagnostic workup and medication interventions. Each of these elements of a delirium care plan, including nonpharmacological and pharmacological interventions to ameliorate symptoms, can be safely provided in any setting of care, including in patients' homes (Irwin et al. 2013).

Patient and Family Education and Support

Supporting the patient and family, via education about the condition and assistance with decision making, is likely to help reduce some of the distress associated with having a loved one experience delirium. Indeed, it is believed that well-supported caregivers can play an important role in helping to prevent, identify, and treat delirium (Rosenbloom-Brunton et al. 2010). Caregivers respond positively to psychoeducational strategies about delirium, which have been shown to boost confidence in surrogate decision making in advanced cancer (Gagnon et al. 2002).

Ensuring Safety

Ensuring safety (for the patient, family, and clinical staff) involves ongoing monitoring of symptoms and management of the environment to reduce potential hazards. Patients with delirium may be prone to wandering, falls, behavioral agitation, or inadvertent self-harm (or harm to others), among other risks (American Psychiatric Association 1999). The delirium care plan can involve a number of interventions aimed at minimizing these risks, described in Table 5–5.

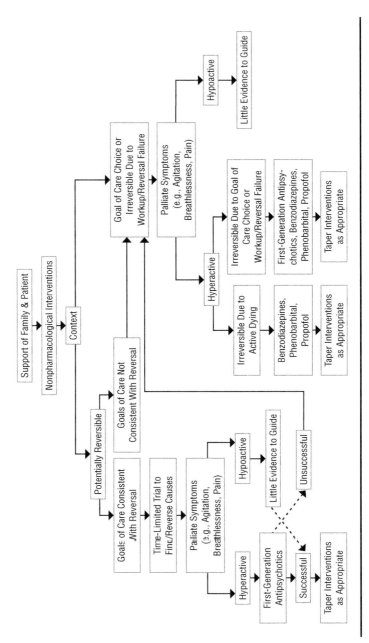

Figure 5–1. Overview of delirium management in the palliative care setting.

Source. Adapted from Irwin et al. 2013.

Table 5–5.   Interventions to improve safety in delirious patients

Monitor frequently: increase surveillance and supervision; consider use of a constant companion.

Ensure access to sensory aids (glasses, hearing aids, etc.); ensure adequate lighting.

Limit access to potentially dangerous items.

Lower beds, pad bed rails, and use mats on floor when appropriate.

Minimize use of lines and cables (e.g., intravenous tubing, Foley catheters, TV and light cables).

Minimize devices that restrict movement.

Source.   Adapted from Irwin et al. 2013.

Addressing the Underlying Cause

In general, efforts to reverse delirium, if desired, are rooted in an understanding of the etiology of the underlying condition, coupled with interventions aimed at reversal of that condition. If the patient's primary disease, baseline functional status, prognosis, and goals for care are consistent with a potentially reversible delirium, then a time-limited and goal-focused diagnostic workup and therapeutic trial to reverse the underlying cause(s) are appropriate. Choices about diagnostic testing should be guided by careful consideration of the potential benefits (in terms of leading to specific, effective, and acceptable interventions), risks, and burdens—and those considerations should be discussed as part of the clarification of goals in developing a plan of care.

If consistent with goals of care and clinical context, an initial workup for potentially reversible causes might include a blood draw (complete metabolic panel, liver panel, ammonia, complete blood count with differential, thyroid-stimulating hormone, and vitamins), blood cultures, a urinalysis, a chest X ray, or an abdominal series to investigate constipation. If these fail to identify any target for reversal, a second-pass workup could include head imaging, electroencephalography, and cerebrospinal fluid analysis.

Ameliorating Symptoms

Nonpharmacological Interventions

Of the strategies aimed at symptom management, nonpharmacological approaches, listed in Table 5–6, are a recommended part of every care plan for delirium in any setting, including palliative care (Breitbart and Alici 2012; Bush et al. 2014; Inouye et al. 2014b; Irwin et al. 2013; LeGrand 2012). There is broad overlap between the multicomponent prevention strategies (described earlier in the "Prevention" section) and the nonpharmacological approaches to ameliorating symptoms, which are both aimed at addressing the many different environmental contributors to delirium, such as changes in sleep-wake cycle, immobility, dehydration, disorientation, and barriers to communication. Nonpharmacological interventions, although frequently underused or overlooked, involve minimal expense and little risk of harm.

Pharmacological Interventions

A sizable number of studies have examined drug treatment approaches to symptom management in delirium. Unfortunately, data of the highest quality—for example, randomized, double-blind, placebo-controlled trials—do not exist, and other results have been inconsistent or of limited generalizability to the palliative care population. No medications have been approved by the U.S. Food and Drug Administration (FDA) for the treatment of delirium. Perhaps unsurprisingly, a wide range of opinion exists regarding the roles for medication in the management of delirium (Agar et al. 2008), with some experts even recently advocating against medication use entirely, given inconsistent data about effectiveness and clear risks of harm (Inouye et al. 2014a). Nonetheless, and notwithstanding the limited availability of high-quality evidence, recent systematic reviews and expert opinion do provide consensus about medication use in delirium (Breitbart and Alici 2012; Bush et al. 2014; Irwin et al. 2013; LeGrand 2012). The pharmacological strategies presented in this section are broadly consistent with the most recent reviews and opinion, and they derive from an evidence-based, expert-consensus approach to the roles (and limitations) of medication for the management of symptoms associated with delirium in palliative care settings.

Given the limited strength of existing evidence, and the significant consequences associated with delirium in seriously ill patients, the importance of

Table 5–6.   Nonpharmacological strategies in the management of delirium

Engage patients in mentally stimulating activities.

Provide frequent orientation (to place and time, to staff, etc.).

Provide familiar materials.

Minimize overstimulation (with TV, loud music, etc.).

Use family or volunteers as constant companions; encourage staff to sit with the patient while documenting.

Provide ambient natural light or soft lighting.

Optimize sleep: provide warm milk, massage, warm blankets; use relaxation tapes; minimize interruption.

Ensure that patients have access to sensory aids (glasses, hearing aids, etc.).

Ensure that patients have good nutrition and effective bowel and bladder care.

Monitor fluid intake; rehydrate with oral fluids containing salt (e.g., soups, sports drinks, red vegetable juices).

Encourage mobility as tolerated.

Minimize use of physical restraints (use only as last resort to temporarily ensure safety; only until less restrictive interventions are possible).

Source.   Adapted from Irwin et al. 2013.

careful communication with patients and families cannot be overstated. Echoing the discussion above regarding goals of care, any conversation about medication use in delirium should take note of the particular clinical context and prognosis, acknowledge the absence of certainty about the potential effects (good and bad) of medications, and be mindful of the degree of suffering and goals of care for the patient and family.

Medication options for symptom management in delirium are provided in Table 5–7. Antipsychotic medications and benzodiazepines are the main choices available, and several other sedative-hypnotic agents (e.g., barbiturates or propofol) may have a limited role, as discussed later in this section. Although drugs from other classes (e.g., opioids, cholinesterase inhibitors, psychostimulants) have been tried as well, there is very little evidence to support their regular use in managing delirium in palliative care, and they should not

Table 5–7.   Drug treatments for symptom management in delirium

Drug by class	Suggested dosing, titration	Recommended prn interval (based on time to C_{max})	Recommended ATC interval (based on half-life)	Notes
Antipsychotics				Recommended in hyperactive delirium, reversible or irreversible. Data do not support efficacy of one agent over another; choose based on side effects, routes, cost, etc.
Haloperidol	1–2 mg PO q 60 min prn agitation Then use titration strategy[a] to establish prn and ATC doses	PO/PR: 60 min SC/IM: 30 min IV: 15 min	bid/tid	Max dose ~100 mg/day Available routes: PO (tabs, liq), PR, SC, IM, IV
Chlorpromazine	25–5 mg PO q 60 min prn agitation Then use titration strategy[a]	PO/PR: 60 min SC/IM: 30 min IV: 15 min	bid/tid	Max dose ~2,000 mg/day Available routes: PO, PR, SC (caustic), IM, IV
Olanzapine	2.5 mg PO q 60 min prn agitation Then use titration strategy[a]	PO: 60 min IM: 30 min	Daily/bid	Max dose ~40 mg/day Available routes: PO (tabs, ODT), IM

Table 5–7.   Drug treatments for symptom management in delirium (*continued*)

Drug by class	Suggested dosing, titration	Recommended prn interval (based on time to C_{max})	Recommended ATC interval (based on half-life)	Notes
Antipsychotics (*continued*)				
Risperidone	0.5 mg PO q 60 min prn agitation Then use titration strategy[a]	PO/PR: 60 min IM: 30 min	Daily/bid	Max dose ~ 16 mg/day Available routes: PO (tabs, liq, ODT)
Quetiapine	25 mg PO q 60 min prn agitation Then use titration strategy[a]	PO/PR: 60 min	bid/tid	Max dose ~ 800 mg/day Available routes: PO (tabs)
Benzodiazepines				Recommended in 1) irreversible delirium, especially with signs of active dying; 2) alcohol or benzodiazepine withdrawal delirium; and 3) severe behavioral agitation. Patients receiving long-term benzodiazepine therapy (e.g., for anxiety) may be refractory to control of agitation with benzodiazepines.

Table 5–7.   Drug treatments for symptom management in delirium (*continued*)

Drug by class	Suggested dosing, titration	Recommended prn interval (based on time to C_{max})	Recommended ATC interval (based on half-life)	Notes
Benzodiazepines (continued)				
Lorazepam	1–2 mg PO q 60 min prn agitation Then use titration strategy[a]	PO/PR: 60 min SC/IM: 30 min IV: 15 min	bid	Max dose ~40 mg/day Available routes: PO (tabs, liq), PR, SC, IM, IV
Midazolam	0.1–0.2 mg/kg SC loading dose Then repeat q 30 min prn agitation Then give 25% of the total dose needed to control symptoms as a continuous SC infusion	SC/IM: 30 min IV: 15 min	Continuous infusion	Max dose ~240 mg/day Available routes: PO (liq), SC, IM, IV
Other sedatives				Generally reserved for control of severe agitation that is refractory to all other measures. Requires consultation with expert in palliative medicine.

Table 5–7.   Drug treatments for symptom management in delirium (*continued*)

Drug by class	Suggested dosing, titration	Recommended prn interval (based on time to C_{max})	Recommended ATC interval (based on half-life)	Notes
Other sedatives (*continued*)				
Phenobarbital	PO/PR: 30–120 mg/day, divided bid/tid SC/IV: 10–30 mg/kg loading dose Then give 20–100 mg/hr continuous SC/IV infusion	PO/PR: 10 hr SC/IM: 2 hr IV: 30 min	bid/tid Continuous infusion	Max dose ~2,400 mg/day Available routes: PO (tabs, liq), PR, SC, IV Consider infusion if prn IM or SC dose requirements exceed injection capacity
Propofol	1 mg/kg/hr IV starting dose Then increase by 0.5 mg/kg q 15 min until symptom control	IV: 1–2 min	Continuous infusion	Max dose ~12 mg/kg/hr Available routes: IV Effective dose usually <6 mg/kg/hr

Note.   No drug treatments have U.S. Food and Drug Administration approval for the management of delirium. Dosing guidelines reflect a general initial strategy based on the clinical experience of the authors and current drug references (Micromedex DRUGDEX 2014). Local experts and other resources should be consulted for specific concerns (e.g., dosing strategies in incomplete responders, or dose adjustments in hepatic/renal insufficiency). ATC=around the clock; bid=twice daily; IM=intramuscular; IV=intravenous; max=maximum; ODT=orally disintegrating tablet; PO=per oral; PR=per rectum; prn=as needed; q=every; SC=subcutaneous; C_{max}=maximum plasma concentration; tid=three times daily.
aSee "Titration Strategy" subsection in this chapter, and Figure 5–2.

Source.   Adapted from Irwin et al. 2013.

be used for this purpose (Breitbart and Alici 2012). Table 5–8 provides an overview of the therapeutic effects of antipsychotics, benzodiazepines, and (for comparison) opioids.

Selecting medication based on reversibility and subtype.   As shown in Figure 5–1, medication selection hinges on the potential for reversibility and the subtype of the delirium:

- *Potentially reversible delirium, hyperactive subtype*—When medications are used, antipsychotics are the first-line choice. Current evidence does not support a clear advantage for any particular agent on the basis of effectiveness. For reasons of cost and ease of administration, haloperidol is frequently recommended as an initial choice.
- *Irreversible delirium, hyperactive subtype*—Antipsychotic medications may be used as the first-line choice; however, use of benzodiazepines may be more appropriate, particularly when there are signs that the patient has entered the final, active phase of the dying process or when sedation is the primary goal. In cases of irreversible delirium in which efforts at symptom relief are refractory to antipsychotic or benzodiazepine therapies, other sedating or anesthetic agents, such as barbiturates or propofol, can be used.
- *Reversible or irreversible delirium, hypoactive subtype*—Limited data are available to guide medication use: antipsychotics may be used, but it is unclear whether or not they are helpful. One approach is to avoid medication use, thereby minimizing the risks resulting from polypharmacy and exposure to adverse effects of medication. On the other hand, in light of recent evidence that even patients with hypoactive delirium can experience perceptual disturbances, careful use of an antipsychotic may be warranted (Boettger and Breitbart 2011; Platt et al. 1994).

Titration strategy.   For behavioral agitation in delirium, rapid and safe relief can be achieved when the titration strategy is informed by knowledge of pharmacokinetics. Figure 5–2 provides a suggested titration strategy for managing agitation in delirium, and Table 5–9 provides sample orders for rapid control of agitation.

Antipsychotics.   Most guidelines recommend the use of an antipsychotic medication, such as haloperidol, for the first-line treatment of hyperactive de-

Table 5–8.   Therapeutic properties of antipsychotics, benzodiazepines, and opioids

Drug class	Antiagitation	Sedation	Amnesia	Antiseizure	Muscle relaxation
Antipsychotics	✓	✓	✗	–	✗
Benzodiazepines	✓	✓	✓	✓	✓
Opioids	✗	✗	✗	–	✗

Note.   ✓ =has property; ✗ =does not have property; – =has opposite property.
Opioids are provided for comparison; as noted in the text, there is no role for opioids in the management of delirium (see "Pharmacological Interventions" subsection in this chapter). Sedation in opioids is a side effect (not a therapeutic effect), and it is unreliable from person to person and drug to drug.

Source.   Adapted from Irwin et al. 2013.

1. **Select an appropriate drug.**

2. **Determine the as-needed (prn) dose and interval:**
   - If the first prn dose does not control target symptoms by the time it has reached maximum plasma concentration (C_{max}), the effectiveness of that administration will not improve with time.
   - Give repeat prn doses on an interval determined by the medication's time to C_{max}, until symptom control is achieved or side effects emerge.
   - If side effects emerge, reduce dose to the last effective dose without side effects, or change medication.
   - For ongoing control of breakthrough agitation, make additional doses available prn, on the interval determined by the time to C_{max}, at the dose that was previously effective.

3. **Determine the around-the-clock (ATC) dose and interval:**
   - Once symptoms are controlled, provide the total dose used in the last 24 hours as a divided ATC dose, based on an interval determined by the half-life ($t_{1/2}$).

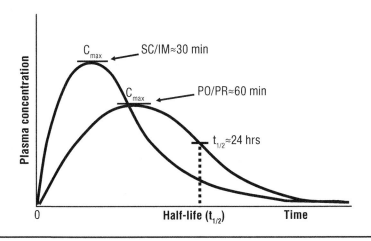

Figure 5–2.   Titration strategy for rapid, rational management of agitation in delirium.   No drug treatments have U.S. Food and Drug Administration approval for the management of delirium. See text for guidance regarding selection of drug. See Table 5–9 for sample orders. The chart refers to all drugs with first-order kinetics. IM = intramuscular; PO = per oral; PR = per rectum; SC = subcutaneous.

Source.   Adapted from Irwin et al. 2013.

Table 5–9. Sample orders for rapid management of delirium

Potentially reversible delirium

Haloperidol	Chlorpromazine
To control:	To control:
• 1 mg SC or IM q 30 min prn agitation.	• 50 mg PO, PR, or IV q 60 min prn agitation.
• If 3 doses are not effective, call physician to reassess dose, diagnosis, or drug.	• If 3 doses are not effective, call physician to reassess dose, diagnosis, or drug.
Once controlled:	Once controlled:
• Schedule the total dose used in the last 24 hrs, given once daily or divided q 12 hrs.	• Schedule the total dose used in the last 24 hrs, given once daily or divided q 12 hrs.
• Continue the prn dose that was previously effective.	• Continue the prn dose that was previously effective.
Caution: Do not exceed 100 mg/24 hrs.	*Caution: Do not exceed 2,000 mg/24 hrs.*
	Caution: SC or IM route can be caustic to skin.

Irreversible delirium

Lorazepam	Midazolam
To control:	To control:
• 1 mg SC or IM q 30 min prn agitation.	• 0.2 mg/kg loading dose SC.
• If 3 doses are not effective, call physician to reassess dose, diagnosis, or drug.	• If needed give additional 0.1 mg/kg q 30 min prn agitation.
Once controlled:	Once controlled:
• Schedule the total dose used in the last 24 hrs, given in two divided doses q 12 hrs.	• Start continuous SC infusion, using 25% of total dose needed for symptom control as hourly rate.
• Continue the prn dose that was previously effective.	• Titrate prn dose by 0.1 mg/kg q 30 min as needed.
Caution: Do not exceed 40 mg/24 hrs.	*Caution: If >10 mg/hr needed for symptom control, consider alternative (barbiturate or propofol).*

Table 5–9.   Sample orders for rapid management of delirium *(continued)*

Acute agitation crisis
Consider the following:
• Give haloperidol 2–5 mg once, by safest accessible route (PO, PR, IM, SC, IV).
• Give with diphenhydramine 50–100 mg to protect against EPS and add sedation.
• Give with lorazepam 1–2 mg if additional sedation desired.
• Can mix slowly in a single syringe, in this order: lorazepam → haloperidol → diphenhydramine.
• May repeat every 30 minutes (if IM or SC) until agitation is controlled.

Note.   No drug treatments have U.S. Food and Drug Administration approval for the management of delirium. See text for guidance regarding selection of drug. As-needed (prn) interval and around-the-clock schedule will vary by route of administration (see text). Patients receiving long-term benzodiazepine therapy (e.g., for anxiety) may be refractory to control of agitation with benzodiazepines. Barbiturates or propofol may be necessary (see Table 5–7). EPS=extrapyramidal symptoms; IM=intramuscular; IV=intravenous; PO=per oral; PR=per rectum; q=every; SC=subcutaneous.

Source.   Adapted from Irwin et al. 2013.

lirium. Antipsychotics reduce psychosis and agitation, and many also provide some degree of sedation, but they do not provide amnesia, muscle relaxation, or an antiseizure effect (see Table 5–8). Little consistent evidence exists for improved efficacy with the newer agents (atypical, or second-generation, antipsychotics), which are often more expensive and have fewer routes of administration. Instead, agents can be distinguished and chosen on the basis of side-effect profiles, cost, routes of administration, and other factors.

The common adverse effects of antipsychotics include extrapyramidal symptoms, sedation, orthostasis, QTc prolongation, and anticholinergic effects, as detailed in Table 5–10. Of note, lower antipsychotic doses are typically adequate to address the symptoms associated with delirium in seriously ill patients, and dose-related side effects appear to occur less frequently in this population (Jackson and Lipman 2004; Lonergan et al. 2007). When higher doses are required to control symptoms, families are often willing to accept the associated risks in order to achieve the goal of relieving suffering from distressful symptoms.

As detailed in Chapter 6, "Dementia (Major Neurocognitive Disorder)," in 2005 the FDA issued a black box warning for second-generation antipsychotics, which were shown to be associated with an increased risk of mortality when used in the management of dementia-related psychosis in elderly patients (Schneider et al. 2005). A subsequent warning was extended to first-generation antipsychotics as well (Wang et al. 2005). These warnings do not pertain to the use of antipsychotics to manage delirium; whether or not their use is associated with mortality risks in this setting is unknown. In a small nested case-control study of hospitalized elderly patients with delirium, antipsychotic use was not associated with increased mortality (Elie et al. 2009).

Benzodiazepines. Except in a few specific clinical situations (e.g., in the management of alcohol withdrawal, or in a crisis of acute agitation), benzodiazepines should *not* be used as first-line agents in the management of a potentially reversible delirium. As noted earlier in this section on pharmacological interventions, there is an important role, however, for benzodiazepines in irreversible delirium, in particular when there are signs of active dying—that is, when the sedation, amnesia, muscle relaxation, and antiseizure effects (see Table 5–8) can become particularly advantageous. Conversely, many of these same effects account for why benzodiazepines should not be used when

Table 5–10.   Common adverse effects of selected antipsychotic medications

Drug	Anticholinergic (M_1)	Sedation (H_1)	Orthostasis (α_1)	QTc prolongation	EPS (D_2)
Haloperidol	×	✓	×	× (PO); ✓✓ (IV)	✓✓✓
Chlorpromazine	✓✓	✓✓✓	✓	✓✓	✓
Risperidone	×	✓	×	✓	✓✓
Olanzapine	✓✓	✓✓	×	×	✓
Quetiapine	×	✓✓✓	✓	✓	×

Note.   ✓ = relative strength of effect; × = does not have effect; α_1 = α_1-adrenergic receptor; D_2 = dopamine receptor type 2; EPS = extrapyramidal symptoms; H_1 = histamine receptor type 1; IV = intravenous; M_1 = muscarinic receptor type 1; PO = per oral.

Source.   Adapted from Irwin et al. 2013.

the goal involves efforts to reverse the delirium. These agents can contribute to confusion (precipitating or worsening a delirium), increase the risk of falls, create memory problems, and lead to withdrawal syndromes. In patients with irreversible, hyperactive delirium, the benefits of these medications are more likely to outweigh the risks.

Other Agents.   Finally, in an irreversible, hyperactive delirium, when benzodiazepines have failed to control agitation, barbiturates or propofol are sometimes used to provide symptom relief (Lundström et al. 2010).

Conclusions and Key Points

- Delirium is an acute change in mental status, marked by a disturbance of attention and other cognitive deficits, and caused by an underlying physiological condition.

- In patients with a serious or advanced medical illness, delirium is highly prevalent, and it has significant adverse consequences.

- Even in the context of a serious or advanced illness, the causes of delirium can frequently be identified and reversed.

- Management strategies for delirium include providing education and support, ensuring safety, addressing underlying causes, and managing symptoms.

- Clarifying the goals of care, within the context of the patient's functional status and prognosis, is of critical importance in addressing delirium, because it can guide choices about workup and management.

- Nonpharmacological interventions should be part of the care plan in all cases of delirium; pharmacological interventions have utility in certain contexts, based on the subtype of delirium, reversibility, and prognosis and goals of care.

References

Agar M, Currow D, Plummer J, et al: Differing management of people with advanced cancer and delirium by four sub-specialties. Palliat Med 22(5):633–640, 2008 18612029

American Psychiatric Association: Practice guideline for the treatment of patients with delirium. Am J Psychiatry 156(5 Suppl):1–20, 1999 10327941

American Psychiatric Association: Diagnostic and Statistical Manual of Mental Disorders, 5th Edition. Arlington, VA, American Psychiatric Association, 2013

Boettger S, Breitbart W: Phenomenology of the subtypes of delirium: phenomenological differences between hyperactive and hypoactive delirium. Palliat Support Care 9(2):129–135, 2011 24468480

Breitbart W, Alici Y: Agitation and delirium at the end of life: "We couldn't manage him." JAMA 300(24):2898–2910, e1, 2008

Breitbart W, Alici Y: Evidence-based treatment of delirium in patients with cancer. J Clin Oncol 30(11):1206–1214, 2012 22412123

Breitbart W, Gibson C, Tremblay A: The delirium experience: delirium recall and delirium-related distress in hospitalized patients with cancer, their spouses/caregivers, and their nurses. Psychosomatics 43(3):183–194, 2002 12075033

Bruera E, Fainsinger RL, Miller MJ, et al: The assessment of pain intensity in patients with cognitive failure: a preliminary report. J Pain Symptom Manage 7(5):267–270, 1992a 1624813

Bruera E, Miller L, McCallion J, et al: Cognitive failure in patients with terminal cancer: a prospective study. J Pain Symptom Manage 7(4):192–195, 1992b 1517640

Bruera E, Bush SH, Willey J, et al: Impact of delirium and recall on the level of distress in patients with advanced cancer and their family caregivers. Cancer 115(9):2004–2012, 2009 19241420

Bush SH, Kanji S, Pereira JL, et al: Treating an established episode of delirium in palliative care: expert opinion and review of the current evidence base with recommendations for future development. J Pain Symptom Manage 48(2):231–248, 2014 24480529

Casarett DJ, Inouye SK; American College of Physicians–American Society of Internal Medicine End-of-Life Care Consensus Panel: Diagnosis and management of delirium near the end of life. Ann Intern Med 135(1):32–40, 2001 11434730

Cohen MZ, Pace EA, Kaur G, et al: Delirium in advanced cancer leading to distress in patients and family caregivers. J Palliat Care 25(3):164–171, 2009 19824277

Cole MG, Ciampi A, Belzile E, et al: Persistent delirium in older hospital patients: a systematic review of frequency and prognosis. Age Ageing 38(1):19–26, 2009 19017678

Davis DH, Muniz Terrera G, Keage H, et al: Delirium is a strong risk factor for dementia in the oldest-old: a population-based cohort study. Brain 135(Pt 9):2809–2816, 2012 22879644

de la Cruz M, Fan J, Yennu S, et al: The frequency of missed delirium in patients referred to palliative care in a comprehensive cancer center. Support Care Cancer 23(8):2427–2433, 2015 25617070

Elie M, Boss K, Cole MG, et al: A retrospective, exploratory, secondary analysis of the association between antipsychotic use and mortality in elderly patients with delirium. Int Psychogeriatr 21(3):588–592, 2009 19368755

Fang CK, Chen HW, Liu SI, et al: Prevalence, detection and treatment of delirium in terminal cancer inpatients: a prospective survey. Jpn J Clin Oncol 38(1):56–63, 2008 18238881

Gagnon P, Charbonneau C, Allard P, et al: Delirium in advanced cancer: a psychoeducational intervention for family caregivers. J Palliat Care 18(4):253–261, 2002 12611315

Gagnon P, Allard P, Gagnon B, et al: Delirium prevention in terminal cancer: assessment of a multicomponent intervention. Psychooncology 21(2):187–194, 2012 22271539

Hempenius L, van Leeuwen BL, van Asselt DZ, et al: Structured analyses of interventions to prevent delirium. Int J Geriatr Psychiatry 26(5):441–450, 2011 20848577

Hosie A, Davidson PM, Agar M, et al: Delirium prevalence, incidence, and implications for screening in specialist palliative care inpatient settings: a systematic review. Palliat Med 27(6):486–498, 2013 22988044

Inouye SK, Charpentier PA: Precipitating factors for delirium in hospitalized elderly persons. Predictive model and interrelationship with baseline vulnerability. JAMA 275(11):852–857, 1996 8596223

Inouye SK, van Dyck CH, Alessi CA, et al: Clarifying confusion: the Confusion Assessment Method. A new method for detection of delirium. Ann Intern Med 113(12):941–948, 1990 2240918

Inouye SK, Rushing JT, Foreman MD, et al: Does delirium contribute to poor hospital outcomes? A three-site epidemiologic study. J Gen Intern Med 13(4):234–242, 1998 9565386

Inouye SK, Bogardus ST Jr, Charpentier PA, et al: A multicomponent intervention to prevent delirium in hospitalized older patients. N Engl J Med 340(9):669–676, 1999 10053175

Inouye SK, Marcantonio ER, Metzger ED: Doing damage in delirium: the hazards of antipsychotic treatment in elderly persons. Lancet Psychiatry 1(4):312–315, 2014a 25285270

Inouye SK, Westendorp RG, Saczynski JS: Delirium in elderly people. Lancet 383(9920): 911–922, 2014b 23992774

Irwin SA, Pirrello RD, Hirst JM, et al: Clarifying delirium management: practical, evidence-based, expert recommendations for clinical practice. J Palliat Med 16(4): 423–435, 2013 23480299

Jackson KC, Lipman AG: Drug therapy for delirium in terminally ill patients. Cochrane Database Syst Rev (2):CD004770, 2004 15106261

Kiely DK, Marcantonio ER, Inouye SK, et al: Persistent delirium predicts greater mortality. J Am Geriatr Soc 57(1):55–61, 2009 19170790

Lawlor PG, Gagnon B, Mancini IL, et al: Occurrence, causes, and outcome of delirium in patients with advanced cancer: a prospective study. Arch Intern Med 160(6):786–794, 2000 10737278

LeGrand SB: Delirium in palliative medicine: a review. J Pain Symptom Manage 44(4): 583–594, 2012 22682074

Leonard M, Raju B, Conroy M, et al: Reversibility of delirium in terminally ill patients and predictors of mortality. Palliat Med 22(7):848–854, 2008 18755829

Leonard MM, Nekolaichuk C, Meagher DJ, et al: Practical assessment of delirium in palliative care. J Pain Symptom Manage 48(2):176–190, 2014 24766745

Leslie DL, Inouye SK: The importance of delirium: economic and societal costs. J Am Geriatr Soc 59(Suppl 2):S241–S243, 2011 22091567

Leslie DL, Zhang Y, Holford TR, et al: Premature death associated with delirium at 1-year follow-up. Arch Intern Med 165(14):1657–1662, 2005 16043686

Lonergan E, Britton AM, Luxenberg J, et al: Antipsychotics for delirium. Cochrane Database Syst Rev (2):CD005594, 2007 17443602

Lundström S, Twycross R, Mihalyo M, et al: Propofol. J Pain Symptom Manage 40(3):466–470, 2010 20816571

Massie MJ, Holland J, Glass E: Delirium in terminally ill cancer patients. Am J Psychiatry 140(8):1048–1050, 1983 6869591

McNicoll L, Pisani MA, Zhang Y, et al: Delirium in the intensive care unit: occurrence and clinical course in older patients. J Am Geriatr Soc 51(5):591–598, 2003 12752832

Meagher D, Moran M, Raju B, et al: A new data-based motor subtype schema for delirium. J Neuropsychiatry Clin Neurosci 20(2):185–193, 2008 18451189

Micromedex DRUGDEX (Internet database). Ann Arbor, MI, Truven Health Analytics, 2014. Available at: www.micromedexsolutions.com. Subscription required to view.

Morita T, Tei Y, Tsunoda J, et al: Underlying pathologies and their associations with clinical features in terminal delirium of cancer patients. J Pain Symptom Manage 22(6):997–1006, 2001 11738162

Namba M, Morita T, Imura C, et al: Terminal delirium: families' experience. Palliat Med 21(7):587–594, 2007 17942497

O'Mahony R, Murthy L, Akunne A, et al; Guideline Development Group: Synopsis of the National Institute for Health and Clinical Excellence guideline for prevention of delirium. Ann Intern Med 154(11):746–751, 2011 21646557

Peterson JF, Pun BT, Dittus RS, et al: Delirium and its motoric subtypes: a study of 614 critically ill patients. J Am Geriatr Soc 54(3):479–484, 2006 16551316

Platt MM, Breitbart W, Smith M, et al: Efficacy of neuroleptics for hypoactive delirium. J Neuropsychiatry Clin Neurosci 6(1):66–67, 1994 7908548

Reston JT, Schoelles KM: In-facility delirium prevention programs as a patient safety strategy: a systematic review. Ann Intern Med 158(5 Pt 2):375–380, 2013 23460093

Rosenbloom-Brunton DA, Henneman EA, Inouye SK: Feasibility of family participation in a delirium prevention program for hospitalized older adults. J Gerontol Nurs 36(9):22–33, quiz 34–35, 2010 20438016

Ross CA, Peyser CE, Shapiro I, et al: Delirium: phenomenologic and etiologic subtypes. Int Psychogeriatr 3(2):135–147, 1991 1811769

Ryan K, Leonard M, Guerin S, et al: Validation of the Confusion Assessment Method in the palliative care setting. Palliat Med 23(1):40–45, 2009 19010967

Schneider LS, Dagerman KS, Insel P: Risk of death with atypical antipsychotic drug treatment for dementia: meta-analysis of randomized placebo-controlled trials. JAMA 294(15):1934–1943, 2005 16234500

Spiller JA, Keen JC: Hypoactive delirium: assessing the extent of the problem for inpatient specialist palliative care. Palliat Med 20(1):17–23, 2006 16482754

Stagno D, Gibson C, Breitbart W: The delirium subtypes: a review of prevalence, phenomenology, pathophysiology, and treatment response. Palliat Support Care 2(2):171–179, 2004 16594247

Tucker R, Nichols A: UNIPAC 4: Managing Non-Pain Symptoms. UNIPAC Self Study Program, 4th Edition. Edited by Storey CP Jr. Glenview, IL, American Academy of Hospice and Palliative Medicine, 2012. Available at: http://www.aahpm.org/resources/default/unipac-4th-edition.html. Accessed July 20, 2015.

Wang PS, Schneeweiss S, Avorn J, et al: Risk of death in elderly users of conventional vs atypical antipsychotic medications. N Engl J Med 353(22):2335–2341, 2005 16319382

Witlox J, Eurelings LS, de Jonghe JF, et al: Delirium in elderly patients and the risk of postdischarge mortality, institutionalization, and dementia: a meta-analysis. JAMA 304(4):443–451, 2010 20664045

Wong CL, Holroyd-Leduc J, Simel DL, et al: Does this patient have delirium? Value of bedside instruments. JAMA 304(7):779–786, 2010 20716741

Additional Resources

Breitbart W, Lawlor PG, Friedlander M: Delirium in the terminally ill, in Handbook of Psychiatry in Palliative Medicine, 2nd Edition. Edited by Chochinov HM, Breitbart W. New York, Oxford University Press, 2009, pp 81–100

Education in Palliative and End-of-Life-Care for Oncology (EPEC-Oncology). Module 3g: Delirium. Available at: http://www.cancer.gov/cancertopics/cancerlibrary/epeco. Accessed July 20, 2015.

ICU Delirium and Cognitive Impairment Study Group. Web site at: http://icu-delirium.org.

Irwin SA, Buckholz GT, Hirst JM, et al: Recognizing and managing delirium, in Principles and Practice of Palliative Care and Supportive Oncology, 4th Edition. Edited by Berger A, Shuster JL, Von Roenn JH. Philadelphia, PA, Lippincott Williams & Wilkins, 2013, pp 529–542

Trzepacz PT, Meagher DJ, Leonard M: Delirium, in Textbook of Psychosomatic Medicine, 2nd Edition. Edited by Levenson JL. Arlington, VA, American Psychiatric Publishing, 2011, pp 71–114

Tucker RO, Nichols AC: UNIPAC 4: Managing Non-Pain Symptoms. UNIPAC Self Study Program, 4th Edition. Edited by Storey CP Jr. Glenview, IL, American Academy of Hospice and Palliative Medicine, 2012. Available at: http://www.aahpm.org/resources/default/unipac-4th-edition.html. Accessed July 20, 2015.

Center to Advance Palliative Care, Fast Facts

Altman RA, Milbrandt E, Arnold RM: Fast Fact #160: Screening for ICU delirium. Available at: https://www.capc.org/fast-facts/160-screening-icu-delirium/. Accessed July 23, 2015.

Billings AJ, Quijada E: Fast Fact #60: Pharmacologic management of delirium: update on newer agents. Available at: https://www.capc.org/fast-facts/60-pharmacologic-management-delirium-update-newer-agents/. Accessed July 23, 2015.

Weissman DE, Roseille DA: Fast Fact #1: Diagnosis and treatment of terminal delirium. Available at: https://www.capc.org/fast-facts/1-diagnosis-and-treatment-terminal-delirium/. Accessed July 23, 2015.

PART III

Other Common Psychiatric Conditions

6

Dementia (Major Neurocognitive Disorder)

Chapter Overview

Dementia can be both a terminal disease and a comorbid condition that greatly complicates the care of individuals in palliative care settings. Palliative care providers frequently struggle with various issues surrounding the care of patients with dementia, including decisions about whether and when to discontinue medication, how to manage psychosis and challenging behaviors, how to support caregivers who experience loss over a prolonged period before the patient dies, and how to best respect a patient's autonomy as his or her ability to make autonomous decisions slips away. In these areas in particular, psychiatric expertise can enhance the care of patients with dementia in palliative care settings. Some of these issues are pursued more generally in other chapters in this text, but this chapter focuses on their application to the care of patients with dementia.

Dementia refers to a broad range of disorders—Alzheimer's disease being the most common and most familiar—that have in common the feature of progressive cognitive decline and functional impairment. Dementias are often comorbid with other diseases that may be the focus of attention in palliative care. Even when dementia is not severe, cognitive impairments can pose a significant barrier to a patient's ability to adhere to complex treatment plans for other diseases, thus making treatment more difficult and increasing the likelihood of poorer outcomes (Brauner et al. 2000). In a large cohort study in the primary care setting, for example, the presence of mild or moderate dementia was a significant risk for mortality, independent of other mortality risk factors (Sachs et al. 2011). In an advanced stage, dementia can be a terminal disease and can be the main focus of intervention in palliative care or hospice settings. Evidence suggests that palliative care services improve the quality of care near the end of life for patients with advanced dementia (Miller et al. 2012; Shega et al. 2008), and surveys reveal an expansion of hospice use for this population since 2000 (Miller et al. 2010). Nonetheless, difficulties with prognostication, poor recognition of when dementia has reached an advanced stage, and policy barriers appear to contribute to underutilization of hospice and palliative care services for patients with advanced dementia (Mitchell et al. 2012).

Epidemiology and Consequences

Epidemiology

Dementia is very common in the United States and other developed countries, and prevalence climbs steeply with advancing age. In 2014, it was estimated that 5.2 million Americans had Alzheimer's disease (the most common form of dementia), including one in nine adults ages 65 years and older, and nearly one-third of adults ages 85 years and older (Alzheimer's Association 2014). Due to the pace of growth of the older-age segment of the U.S. population, the number of adults with Alzheimer's disease is projected to reach 7.1 million by 2025 and 13.8 million by 2050 (Hebert et al. 2003). In 2009, Alzheimer's disease was the sixth leading cause of death in the United States, which is likely an underestimate due to difficulty distinguishing between "dying with" and "dying from" Alzheimer's disease (Tejada-Vera 2013).

Consequences

The clinical course of advanced dementia is characterized by a protracted period of progressive and severe debility, associated with major impairments in quality of life (Mitchell et al. 2009), high levels of caregiver stress (Fonareva and Oken 2014), and significant economic costs (Alzheimer's Association 2014). Mitchell et al. (2009) published a prospective cohort study of more than 300 nursing home residents with advanced dementia. Over 18 months of surveillance, pneumonia (41.1%), febrile episodes (44.5%), and eating problems (85.8%) were common complications of care. Patients frequently experienced distressful symptoms, including dyspnea, pain, pressure ulcers, aspiration, and agitation, and in the last 3 months of life, over 40% of them underwent at least one burdensome intervention such as hospitalization, parenteral therapy, or tube feeding. Overall, 6-month mortality in advanced dementia appears to be approximately 25%, although estimates vary based on the setting and definition used for advanced dementia (Mitchell et al. 2004).

Definitions and Classification

In the fifth edition of the *Diagnostic and Statistical Manual of Mental Disorders* (DSM-5), the American Psychiatric Association (2013) classifies dementing illnesses under the umbrella of neurocognitive disorders.[1] Although specific dementias are differentiated on the basis of etiology and symptomatology, all neurocognitive disorders share the feature of an acquired cognitive decline. Cognition is a multifaceted construct, and the domains of cognitive performance impacted by neurocognitive disorders include complex attention, executive function, learning, memory, language, perceptual motor skill, and social cognition. As shown in Table 6–1, neurocognitive disorders are further classified in DSM-5 as mild and major, according to the severity of cognitive decline and whether or not the deficits interfere with functional capacity. In mild neurocognitive disorders, measurable cognitive deficits are present in at least one domain, but the impairments do not interfere with activities of everyday independence. As cognitive deficits worsen, the patient's ability to maintain control over his or her own care erodes. Patients with advanced dementia typically suffer profound memory impairment (sometimes manifested by an inability to recognize loved ones), severe language deficits (e.g., minimal

---

[1]Delirium, described in Chapter 5, "Delirium," is also included in this diagnostic class, but it is distinguished from dementia primarily by its temporal pattern (its onset is acute or subacute) and its etiology (it results from an underlying physiological condition).

Table 6–1.   DSM-5 criteria for major and mild neurocognitive disorder

DSM-5 criteria for major neurocognitive disorder	DSM-5 criteria for mild neurocognitive disorder
A. Evidence of significant cognitive decline from a previous level of performance in one or more cognitive domains (complex attention, executive function, learning and memory, language, perceptual-motor, or social cognition) based on:	A. Evidence of modest cognitive decline from a previous level of performance in one or more cognitive domains (complex attention, executive function, learning and memory, language, perceptual-motor, or social cognition) based on:
1. Concern of the individual, a knowledgeable informant, or the clinician that there has been a significant decline in cognitive function; and	1. Concern of the individual, a knowledgeable informant, or the clinician that there has been a mild decline in cognitive function; and
2. A substantial impairment in cognitive performance, preferably documented by standardized neuropsychological testing or, in its absence, another quantified clinical assessment.	2. A modest impairment in cognitive performance, preferably documented by standardized neuropsychological testing or, in its absence, another quantified clinical assessment.
B. The cognitive deficits interfere with independence in everyday activities (i.e., at a minimum, requiring assistance with complex instrumental activities of daily living such as paying bills or managing medications).	B. The cognitive deficits do not interfere with capacity for independence in everyday activities (i.e., complex instrumental activities of daily living such as paying bills or managing medications are preserved, but greater effort, compensatory strategies, or accommodation may be required).
C. The cognitive deficits do not occur exclusively in the context of a delirium.	C. The cognitive deficits do not occur exclusively in the context of a delirium.

Table 6–1.   DSM-5 criteria for major and mild neurocognitive disorder *(continued)*

DSM-5 criteria for major neurocognitive disorder *(cont'd)*	DSM-5 criteria for mild neurocognitive disorder *(cont'd)*
D. The cognitive deficits are not better explained by another mental disorder (e.g., major depressive disorder, schizophrenia).	D. The cognitive deficits are not better explained by another mental disorder (e.g., major depressive disorder, schizophrenia).
Specify whether due to: Alzheimer's disease Frontotemporal lobar degeneration Lewy body disease Vascular disease Traumatic brain injury Substance/medication use HIV infection Prion disease Parkinson's disease Huntington's disease Another medical condition Multiple etiologies Unspecified	*Specify* whether due to: Alzheimer's disease Frontotemporal lobar degeneration Lewy body disease Vascular disease Traumatic brain injury Substance/medication use HIV infection Prion disease Parkinson's disease Huntington's disease Another medical condition Multiple etiologies Unspecified
Specify: **Without behavioral disturbance:** If the cognitive disturbance is not accompanied by any clinically significant behavioral disturbance. **With behavioral disturbance** *(specify disturbance)*: If the cognitive disturbance is accompanied by a clinically significant behavioral disturbance (e.g., psychotic symptoms, mood disturbance, agitation, apathy, or other behavioral symptoms).	*Specify:* **Without behavioral disturbance:** If the cognitive disturbance is not accompanied by any clinically significant behavioral disturbance. **With behavioral disturbance** *(specify disturbance)*: If the cognitive disturbance is accompanied by a clinically significant behavioral disturbance (e.g., psychotic symptoms, mood disturbance, agitation, apathy, or other behavioral symptoms).

Table 6–1.   DSM-5 criteria for major and mild neurocognitive disorder (*continued*)

DSM-5 criteria for major neurocognitive disorder (*cont'd*)

Specify current severity:

Mild: Difficulties with instrumental activities of daily living
   (e.g., housework, managing money).

Moderate: Difficulties with basic activities of daily living
   (e.g., feeding, dressing).

Severe: Fully dependent.

Note.   Criteria set above contains only the diagnostic criteria and specifiers; refer to DSM-5 for the full criteria set, including coding and reporting procedures.

Source.   DSM-5 criteria for major and mild neurocognitive disorder reprinted from *Diagnostic and Statistical Manual of Mental Disorders*, 5th Edition. Washington, DC, American Psychiatric Association, 2013, pp. 602–606. Used with permission. Copyright © 2013 American Psychiatric Association.

vocabulary), incontinence, and complete functional dependence. Table 6–2 describes the specific dementias most commonly encountered in palliative care settings; they include dementias due to Alzheimer's disease, Lewy body disease, vascular disease, frontotemporal lobar degeneration, Parkinson's disease, and HIV infection (Lipton and Weiner 2009).

Assessment

Screening for Cognitive Impairment

Major neurocognitive disorders are generally diagnosed on the basis of a clinical examination, often with expert consultation by a neurologist and/or geriatric psychiatrist. For the generalist, a number of screening instruments, described in Table 6–3, are available to assist in the objective assessment of cognition; the results may serve as a trigger for further assessment of dementia. For example, the Mini-Mental State Examination (MMSE; Folstein et al. 1975) is widely used and has been thoroughly studied. A recent systematic review reported that the MMSE has good psychometric properties among patients with suspected dementia in primary care settings, although it appears to lack sensitivity in early dementia (Velayudhan et al. 2014). The Montreal Cognitive Assessment (Nasreddine et al. 2005) is reported to have better sensitivity, relative to the MMSE, in patients with mild cognitive deficits (Smith et al. 2007). In two independent systematic reviews of dementia screening tools, the General Practitioner Assessment of Cognition (Brodaty et al. 2002), the Mini-Cognitive Assessment Tool (Borson et al. 2003), and the Memory Impairment Screen (Buschke et al. 1999) were found to be suitable for routine dementia screening in primary care settings, based on their ease of use and psychometric properties (Brodaty et al. 2006; Milne et al. 2008).

Notably, although these instruments have utility in providing objective measures of some domains of cognition, the role of universal cognitive screening (e.g., as a strategy for primary or secondary prevention) is unclear. A systematic review for the U.S. Preventive Services Task Force found that studies of screening instruments were highly heterogeneous and failed to link test performance to meaningful clinical or societal outcomes (Lin et al. 2013). Nonetheless, the use of such tests, along with a thorough clinical examination, can help the practitioner decide whether further, more detailed neuropsychiatric assessment and workup should be pursued.

Table 6–2. Neurocognitive disorders commonly encountered in palliative care

Etiology	Features
Alzheimer's disease	Most common cause of dementia Central feature is memory impairment, which occurs early Language and visuospatial abilities impacted early in course; behavioral and executive dysfunction tend to present later in the disease
Lewy body disease	Second most common form of dementia Central feature is progressive cognitive decline Early signs are deficits in attention, executive function, visuospatial function Memory impairments tend to present later in the disease Core features: fluctuations in alertness and cognition (60%–80%), visual hallucinations (50%–75%), parkinsonism (80%–90%) Suggestive features: rapid eye movement (REM) sleep behavior disorder, neuroleptic sensitivity
Vascular dementia	Includes multi-infarct dementia and vascular cognitive impairment Results from cerebral vascular pathology; can occur with or without clinically apparent stroke Some studies cite this as the second most common form of dementia Central feature is heterogeneous cognitive impairment resulting from vascular insults Clinical deficits correspond to locations of vascular pathology "Mixed dementia"—dementia resulting from combined Alzheimer's and vascular disease
Frontotemporal dementia	Includes Pick's disease and frontal lobe dementia Results from focal degeneration of the frontal and/or temporal lobes Often marked by personality changes and disinhibition Progressive aphasia and heterogeneous cognitive deficits are present later in the disease Onset in late 50s to early 60s

Table 6–2.   Neurocognitive disorders commonly encountered in palliative care *(continued)*

Etiology	Features
Parkinson's disease dementia	Dementia is a common feature of Parkinson's disease (40%) Results from loss of cholinergic and dopaminergic neurons; anticholinergic agents can negatively impact cognitive function Central features are impairments in executive function, visuospatial function, and verbal memory
HIV-associated dementia	Results from HIV infection affecting deep gray matter brain structures Marked by broad impairments in executive function, attention, working memory, learning, information processing, and psychomotor speed; apathy and irritability may also be features Impairments can wax and wane, depending on status of HIV management

Source.   Adapted from Lipton and Weiner 2009.

Differential Diagnosis

From the standpoint of potential psychiatric involvement in dementia management in palliative care settings, there are several pertinent issues related to differential diagnosis of cognitive disorders. Broadly, ensuring an accurate diagnosis in a patient with cognitive impairment is important because treatments can differ widely. For example, a critical distinction should be made between most dementias and those due to Lewy body or Parkinson's disease, with respect to the use of antipsychotic medication. Patients with dementia due to Lewy body disease or Parkinson's disease can be highly sensitive to the adverse effects of dopamine receptor antagonists, including many antipsychotics and some antiemetics. Such drugs should be avoided altogether or used with caution in these two groups, yet the same agents may be useful in some circumstances in patients with other neurocognitive disorders. As another example, delirium is highly prevalent in palliative care patients, including those with dementia. The fact that delirium is sometimes mistaken for a dementing illness is problematic because the approach to management differs substantially between the two conditions. (Delirium, detailed in Chapter 5, is marked by an acute or subacute onset, results from an underlying medical cause, and may have a fluctuating course—all of which are helpful in differentiating it from dementia.)

Table 6–3.   Cognitive function screening instruments

Instrument	Description
Mini-Mental State Examination (Folstein et al. 1975)	Most widely used brief screening tool for cognitive impairment (Shulman et al. 2006) Approximately 10 minutes to administer 30 points, testing orientation, registration, attention and calculation, recall, and language Good psychometric properties overall, but appears to lack sensitivity in early dementia (Velayudhan et al. 2014)
Montreal Cognitive Assessment (Nasreddine et al. 2005)	Approximately 10 minutes to administer 30 points, testing short-term memory, visuospatial skill, executive function, attention, concentration, working memory, language, and orientation Good sensitivity for detecting mild cognitive impairment (Velayudhan et al. 2014) Available online with instructions on administration: www.mocatest.org
Mini-Cognitive Assessment Tool (Borson et al. 2003)	Approximately 3 minutes to administer Combines three-item word memory and clock drawing Requires little training to administer and interpret Solid performance characteristics in a wide variety of patients Recommended by two independent reviews for use in primary care setting (Brodaty et al. 2006; Milne et al. 2008)
General Practitioner Assessment of Cognition (Brodaty et al. 2002)	Approximately 5 minutes to administer Combines time orientation, clock drawing, report of recent event, and word recall Includes optional assessment from caregiver or informant Recommended by two independent reviews for use in primary care setting (Brodaty et al. 2006; Milne et al. 2008)

Table 6–3. Cognitive function screening instruments *(continued)*

Instrument	Description
Memory Impairment Screen (Buschke et al. 1999)	Approximately 4 minutes to administer Uses four items to test free and cued recall Moderately low sensitivity, but high specificity, and performance may not be affected by age or education (Velayudhan et al. 2014) Recommended by two independent reviews for use in primary care setting (Brodaty et al. 2006; Milne et al. 2008)

Prognostication and Access to Palliative Services

Predicting the course of dementia can be extremely challenging. Unfortunately, late-stage dementia is often associated with poor quality of life and significant caregiver stress, both of which can persist over a long period of time because of the slow progression of the disease. Even in cases of advanced disease, it is notoriously difficult to give accurate prognostic guidance to patients and loved ones, and existing prognostic tools provide only limited assistance in identifying patients who have entered their last 6 months of life, which is the threshold for medical eligibility for hospice care in the United States. These factors likely contribute to underutilization of hospice and palliative care services among patients with advanced dementia.

Table 6–4 provides the current guidelines for eligibility for hospice services for individuals with advanced dementia, from the National Hospice and Palliative Care Organization. In brief, the Medicare hospice benefit requires that patients with dementia have a prognosis of 6 months or less, which is determined in practice by meeting the following two criteria (National Hospice Organization 1996):

1. Must be at stage 7c of the Functional Assessment Staging Test (Reisberg 1988)
2. Must have experienced at least one of the following six medical conditions within the past year: aspiration, urinary tract infection, sepsis, stage 3–4 decubitus ulcers, recurrent fever, or weight loss

Table 6–4.   National Hospice and Palliative Care Organization guidelines for hospice eligibility for dementia

Patients must have reached Stage 7c on the Functional Assessment Staging Test (Reisberg 1988):

1. No cognitive deficits
2. Very mild cognitive deficits (e.g. subjective forgetfulness)
3. Mild cognitive deficits (e.g. decreased job functioning and organizational capacity)
4. Moderate cognitive deficits (e.g. difficulty with complex tasks; deficits with instrumental ADLs)
5. Moderately severe cognitive deficits (e.g. requires supervision with ADLs)
6. Severe cognitive deficits (e.g. severely impaired ADLs; experiencing incontinence)
7. Very severe cognitive deficits
   a. Ability to speak limited to six words
   b. Ability to speak limited to single word
   c. Loss of ambulation
   d. Inability to sit
   e. Inability to smile
   f. Inability to hold up head

Patients must have experienced one of six medical conditions in the past year:

1. Aspiration pneumonia
2. Urinary tract infection, pyelonephritis
3. Sepsis
4. Multiple stage 3–4 decubitus ulcers
5. Recurrent fever
6. Weight loss (>10% over 6 months)

Note.   ADLs=activities of daily living.

Source.   Adapted from National Hospice Organization 1996.

Although patients with this degree of impairment experience poor quality of life, data suggest that these criteria fail to accurately predict 6-month survival (Brown et al. 2013). In fact, patients with severe dementia enrolled in hospice are significantly more likely than those with cancer to survive longer than 6 months—and then to require a face-to-face recertification assessment and potential discharge from hospice (Rothenberg et al. 2014).

Among the alternative strategies for predicting survival, the Advanced Dementia Prognostic Tool (ADEPT; Mitchell et al. 2010a) is perhaps the best studied. The ADEPT score is derived from 12 demographic and clinical domains (e.g., age, weight loss, the presence of pressure ulcers, bowel incontinence), with higher scores associated with a greater risk of death. The ADEPT score appears to be moderately accurate in predicting 6-month survival in nursing home residents with advanced dementia and to be better than the Medicare guidelines in this regard (Mitchell et al. 2010b). Nonetheless, its accuracy overall remains modest, and it is unclear whether these results are generalizable to community-dwelling individuals with advanced dementia.

Hence, even the best prognostic tools are only modestly accurate in predicting 6-month survival, and (more important) quality of life can suffer tremendously long before patients with dementia enter the last 6 months of life. For these reasons, questions have been raised about the arbitrariness of the 6-month restriction, and many experts recommend that goals of care, and not prognosis, ought to guide decisions about access to enhanced palliative care services for patients with advanced dementia (Mitchell et al. 2010a; Passmore 2013; Sokol 2013; Torke et al. 2010).

Management Issues Specific to Psychiatric Palliative Care

In treating patients with dementia in palliative care settings, several management issues often arise for which psychiatric expertise can be particularly valuable; these are pursued in more detail in this section.

Making Decisions About Continuing Medication Therapy

In patients with advanced dementia, as the goals of treatment focus increasingly on comfort, the utility of continued medication therapy is frequently unclear. Many medications that once provided a certain benefit may no longer have a role with respect to achieving comfort-oriented goals in the context of advanced dementia. In this setting, patient-defined goals of care should guide decision making about medication use, and patients should be spared exposure to drugs that are unlikely to advance those goals.

In a 2008 consensus panel survey of geriatricians and palliative medicine specialists, 81 commonly used medications were classified according to their appropriateness in the setting of advanced dementia (Holmes et al. 2008). Broadly, "always appropriate" agents were those that provide an immediate benefit in terms of comfort (e.g., analgesics or laxatives) or safety (e.g., bronchodilators or antiepileptics), whereas drugs that confer benefit through prevention of chronic disease (e.g., lipid-lowering agents) or are immediately toxic (e.g., chemotherapies) were classified as "never appropriate." Of note, the latter class included the cholinesterase inhibitors and the N-methyl-D-aspartate (NMDA) receptor antagonist memantine, both of which are used as "cognitive enhancers" in mild to moderate Alzheimer's disease. Antidepressant and antipsychotic medications were classified as "sometimes appropriate," depending on the indication and context. In addition, other agents of concern include those that can predispose to further cognitive impairment and delirium, such as anticholinergics, opioids, systemic steroids, and benzodiazepines. In a related follow-up study of nursing home patients with advanced dementia, over half the subjects continued to receive medication of questionable benefit (those designated as "never appropriate"), with cholinesterase inhibitors, memantine, and lipid-lowering agents among the most commonly prescribed (Tjia et al. 2014). Notably, hospice enrollment in that study was associated with a significantly reduced likelihood of inappropriate medication use.

Families sometimes experience discomfort around the idea of stopping so-called cognitive-enhancing medications in advanced dementia, so this decision needs to be approached sensitively. Such discussions can trigger concerns that symptoms will worsen or that the disease process will accelerate without continued use of the medication. Similarly, stopping medication that was once believed important can elicit feelings of guilt about "giving up" on a loved one. Communication strategies that anticipate and normalize these concerns, and that focus on the shared goals of ensuring comfort and minimizing harm, are often effective when discussing the discontinuation of inappropriate medication.

Managing Behavioral Disturbances and Psychosis

Neuropsychiatric symptoms are widespread in Alzheimer's disease and most other dementias, and they can range from apathy and depression to frank psychosis (delusions, hallucinations) stereotyped behaviors and vocalizations, disinhibition, behavioral agitation, and aggression. Of these, apathy appears to be the most frequent and persistent across all stages of Alzheimer's disease, but psychotic symptoms and aggressive behavior can become more common with disease progression (Lyketsos et al. 2011). The management of neuropsychiatric symptoms is particularly challenging because such symptoms cause significant suffering in patients and family, nonpharmacological treatments provide only partial relief and are often not practical, and pharmacological interventions are only modestly effective and can be associated with significant harms. In this setting, careful clarification of goals—engaging surrogates in a discussion about trade-offs and tolerance of risks, in particular—is critically important.

Numerous nonpharmacological strategies for managing neuropsychiatric symptoms have been described. Broadly, such interventions can be classified into three groups: 1) those that seek to identify and address unmet needs, 2) those that rely on behavioral strategies, and 3) those aimed at addressing an imbalance between environmental stress and coping reserves. A small 2006 systematic review found some support for nonpharmacological strategies, although results were mixed and data quality was modest (Ayalon et al. 2006). In a larger systematic review in 2012, fewer than half of the studies that met inclusion criteria had positive results on neuropsychiatric symptoms, and the feasibility of implementation in long-term-care settings was questioned (Seitz et al. 2012). Finally, in a small randomized, placebo-controlled trial, a strategy aimed at unmet needs resulted in significant improvements in several domains of agitation (Cohen-Mansfield et al. 2012).

Despite multiple trials, drug therapies have had mixed results in the management of neuropsychiatric symptoms in dementia, and no drug has U.S. Food and Drug Administration (FDA) approval for this indication. Antipsychotic medications have received the most attention, but available evidence suggests that the benefits of antipsychotics in the setting of dementia-related psychosis are likely to be modest at best (Seitz et al. 2013; Steinberg and Lyketsos 2012). The FDA issued a black box warning in 2005 concerning the increased mortality risk with second-generation antipsychotics when used to treat symptoms of psychosis in dementia; the warning was later extended to first-generation antipsychotics as well. The warnings were based on large meta-analyses, showing a small but significant risk of death (primarily from cardiovascular events or pneumonia) for the drugs relative to placebo (Schneider et al. 2005; P.S. Wang et al. 2005). Several subsequent studies have replicated these findings. A large retrospective case control study provided estimates of absolute mortality risk and number needed to harm (NNH) for several antipsychotics: haloperidol appeared to confer the most risk (mortality risk = 3.8%; NNH =

26) and quetiapine the least (mortality risk = 2.0%; NNH = 50), with risperidone and olanzapine falling between these two. Of note, results from this study also suggest a dose-dependent relationship between mortality risk and antipsychotic use (Maust et al. 2015). In the hospice setting, families are often willing to accept these risks if symptom control can be achieved and quality of life for the patient and family can be improved.

Antidepressants have also been studied for their potential role in addressing neuropsychiatric symptoms. In a Cochrane review, Seitz et al. (2011) found six small studies of varying design, two of which reported reductions in agitation (using sertraline and citalopram). More recently, in a multi-site, randomized placebo-controlled, double-blind trial, citalopram was associated with significant reductions in agitation, but titration was limited by adverse effects, including QTc prolongation and cognitive decline (Porsteinsson et al. 2014).

Finally, cholinesterase inhibitors and the NMDA receptor antagonist memantine also have mixed results in the management of neuropsychiatric symptoms. A recent meta-analysis of randomized controlled trials reported some benefit with cholinesterase inhibitors (and none with memantine), but also increased risk of adverse events (J. Wang et al. 2015).

In summary, there is no clear, effective, risk-free intervention for ameliorating neuropsychiatric symptoms in advanced dementia. Environmental and behavioral approaches have shown promise in some settings, yet overall the data quality is low and there are barriers to widespread implementation. Likewise, studies have failed to provide strong support for the effectiveness of drug treatments, which are associated with significant risks.

A recent expert panel (Kales et al. 2014) provided the following guidance regarding the management of neuropsychiatric symptoms:

- Nonpharmacological strategies should be the cornerstone of intervention, using the "DICE" framework: 1) the caregiver Describes problematic behavior, 2) the provider Investigates possible causes, 3) the team Collaborates to create and implement a treatment plan, and 4) the provider Evaluates whether interventions have been safe and effective.
- Psychotropic medication should be considered and used only when reasonable nonpharmacological strategies have been ineffective. In addition, drug treatment may be warranted in any of the following circumstances:

comorbid major depression, psychosis with imminent risk of harm, or aggressive behavior causing risk to the patient or others. Finally, drug treatments should be monitored closely for adverse effects and should be structured in time-limited trials.

Attending to Caregiver Stress

Providing support to caregivers is a major area of focus in palliative care. As a chronic stressor, dementia caregiving, in particular, is known to be associated with adverse health outcomes (Fonareva and Oken 2014; Vitaliano et al. 2003). The symptom domains of dementia and the protracted course of the disease leave caregivers in the position of adapting to ongoing, significant losses on a chronic basis—over the course of years, in many cases. Perhaps unsurprisingly, neuropsychiatric symptoms and perceived poor quality of life in the patient appear to be the factors most closely correlated with caregiver burden and symptoms of depression in dementia caregiving (Mohamed et al. 2010). These findings suggest that attention to promoting quality of life and managing neuropsychiatric symptoms in patients with dementia may have the added benefit of ameliorating caregiver distress. In fact, some evidence suggests that treatment of neuropsychiatric symptoms may reduce caregiver stress (Mohamed et al. 2012), although data are mixed about this (Levy et al. 2012). Palliative care services appear to help alleviate stress in caregivers whose loved ones have dementia (Shega et al. 2008). In a small study of spousal caregivers with Alzheimer's disease, for example, caregivers receiving hospice services were found to exhibit reductions in symptoms of depression and anxiety, relative to those not enrolled in hospice (Irwin et al. 2013).

Supporting Autonomy When Decision-Making Capacity Is in Decline

Progressive cognitive decline undermines autonomous decision making in patients with dementia. As a consequence, family members and clinicians often struggle with uncertainty about whether treatments are consistent with the patient's wishes. Ultimately, such struggles arise from an ethical tension between the obligation to respect autonomy on the one hand, and the duty to protect patients whose capacity for autonomous decision making is impaired on the other. The care of patients with advanced dementia exemplifies the intersection of a number of vexing ethical and clinical issues, for which expertise in psychiatric palliative care is often helpful.

When decision-making capacity is in decline, efforts to support autonomy can perhaps be grouped in two domains: 1) early opportunities to ensure that future care is aligned with the patient's goals and 2) strategies to support surrogate decision making in later stages of disease. Early advance care planning discussions, for example, can help patients to reflect on future priorities of care, including eventual decisions about hospitalization and long-term institutionalization, the use of antibiotics, approaches to nutrition and hydration, and the role of cardiopulmonary resuscitation (CPR) or mechanical ventilation. Early clarification of patients' preferences (i.e., while they still retain decisional capacity) is likely to have the future benefit of helping to unburden family members of uncertainty and distress when they are needed to act as surrogate decision makers (Fritsch et al. 2013; Wendler and Rid 2011). Hence, in the case of dementia, the ongoing process of clarifying goals of care will involve careful attention to educating the patient and family about the expected course of disease, ongoing assessment of decisional capacity, and supporting family members with the tasks of surrogate decision making—all with the aim of providing care that is anchored by respect for the patient's autonomy, even long after the disease has taken away the patient's decisional capacity. Palliative care psychiatrists are in a unique position to facilitate these conversations and thus help patients and their loved ones avoid potentially unwanted interventions as their disease advances.

Conclusions and Key Points

- Dementias are marked by progressive deterioration of cognition, inexorable functional decline, and profound diminishment of quality of life.

- Major neurocognitive disorders are a leading cause of death in the United States, and they can be the main focus of intervention in palliative and hospice care.

- Even the best prognostic tools are only modestly accurate in predicting 6-month survival in dementia. Many experts recommend that goals of care, and not prognosis, ought to guide decisions about access to hospice services.

- In advanced dementia, medications that no longer serve a meaningful clinical goal should be discontinued.

- In advanced dementia, neuropsychiatric symptoms are common and highly distressful to patients, family, and clinicians.

- There are no clearly effective, risk-free interventions for ameliorating neuropsychiatric symptoms. Nonpharmacological strategies are associated with modest benefit, but there are barriers to implementation. Drug treatments are associated with unclear benefit and known risks.

- Early and ongoing clarification of goals is likely to help support autonomy and surrogate decision making as decisional capacity declines in patients with dementia.

- Attention to caregiver distress is an essential component of effective palliative care in patients with advanced dementia.

References

Alzheimer's Association: 2014 Alzheimer's disease facts and figures. Alzheimers Dement 10(2):e47–e92, 2014 24818261

American Psychiatric Association: Diagnostic and Statistical Manual of Mental Disorders, 5th Edition. Arlington, VA, American Psychiatric Association, 2013

Ayalon L, Gum AM, Feliciano L, et al: Effectiveness of nonpharmacological interventions for the management of neuropsychiatric symptoms in patients with dementia: a systematic review. Arch Intern Med 166(20):2182–2188, 2006 17101935

Borson S, Scanlan JM, Chen P, Ganguli M: The Mini-Cog as a screen for dementia: validation in a population-based sample. J Am Geriatr Soc 51(10):1451–1454, 2003 14511167

Brauner DJ, Muir JC, Sachs GA: Treating nondementia illnesses in patients with dementia. JAMA 283(24):3230–3235, 2000 10866871

Brodaty H, Pond D, Kemp NM, et al: The GPCOG: a new screening test for dementia designed for general practice. Am J Geriatr Soc 50(3):530–534, 2002 11943052

Brodaty H, Low LF, Gibson L, et al: What is the best dementia screening instrument for general practitioners to use? Am J Geriatr Psychiatry 14(5):391–400, 2006 16670243

Brown MA, Sampson EL, Jones L, et al: Prognostic indicators of 6-month mortality in elderly people with advanced dementia: a systematic review. Palliat Med 27(5): 389–400, 2013 23175514

Buschke H, Kuslansky G, Katz M, et al: Screening for dementia with the memory impairment screen. Neurology 52(2):231–238, 1999 9932936

Cohen-Mansfield J, Thein K, Marx MS, et al: Efficacy of nonpharmacologic interventions for agitation in advanced dementia: a randomized, placebo-controlled trial. J Clin Psychiatry 73(9):1255–1261, 2012 23059151

Folstein MF, Folstein SE, McHugh PR: "Mini-mental state": a practical method for grading the cognitive state of patients for the clinician. J Psychiatr Res 12(3):189–198, 1975 1202204

Fonareva I, Oken BS: Physiological and functional consequences of caregiving for relatives with dementia. Int Psychogeriatr 26(5):725–747, 2014 24507463

Fritsch J, Petronio S, Helft PR, et al: Making decisions for hospitalized older adults: ethical factors considered by family surrogates. J Clin Ethics 24(2):125–134, 2013 23923811

Hebert LE, Scherr PA, Bienias JL, et al: Alzheimer disease in the U.S. population: prevalence estimates using the 2000 census. Arch Neurol 60(8):1119–1122, 2003 12925369

Holmes HM, Sachs GA, Shega JW, et al: Integrating palliative medicine into the care of persons with advanced dementia: identifying appropriate medication use. J Am Geriatr Soc 56(7):1306–1311, 2008 18482301

Irwin SA, Mausbach BT, Koo D, et al: Association between hospice care and psychological outcomes in Alzheimer's spousal caregivers. J Palliat Med 16(11):1450–1454, 2013 24093721

Kales HC, Gitlin LN, Lyketsos CG; Detroit Expert Panel on Assessment and Management of Neuropsychiatric Symptoms of Dementia: Management of neuropsychiatric symptoms of dementia in clinical settings: recommendations from a multidisciplinary expert panel. J Am Geriatr Soc 62(4):762–769, 2014 24635665

Levy K, Lanctôt KL, Farber SB, et al: Does pharmacological treatment of neuropsychiatric symptoms in Alzheimer's disease relieve caregiver burden? Drugs Aging 29(3):167–179, 2012 22350526

Lin JS, O'Connor E, Rossom RC, et al: Screening for cognitive impairment in older adults: a systematic review for the U.S. Preventive Services Task Force. Ann Intern Med 159(9):601–612, 2013 24145578

Lipton AM, Weiner MF: The American Psychiatric Publishing Textbook of Alzheimer Disease and Other Dementias. Washington, DC, American Psychiatric Publishing, 2009

Lyketsos CG, Carrillo MC, Ryan JM, et al: Neuropsychiatric symptoms in Alzheimer's disease. Alzheimers Dement 7(5):532–539, 2011 21889116

Maust DT, Kim HM, Seyfried LS, et al: Antipsychotics, other psychotropics, and the risk of death in patients with dementia: number needed to harm. JAMA Psychiatry 72(5):438–445, 2015 25786075

Miller SC, Lima JC, Mitchell SL: Hospice care for persons with dementia: the growth of access in U.S. nursing homes. Am J Alzheimers Dis Other Demen 25(8):666–673, 2010 21131673

Miller SC, Lima JC, Looze J, et al: Dying in U.S. nursing homes with advanced dementia: how does health care use differ for residents with, versus without, end-of-life Medicare skilled nursing facility care? J Palliat Med 15(1):43–50, 2012 22175816

Milne A, Culverwell A, Guss R, et al: Screening for dementia in primary care: a review of the use, efficacy and quality of measures. Int Psychogeriatr 20(5):911–926, 2008 18533066

Mitchell SL, Kiely DK, Hamel MB, et al: Estimating prognosis for nursing home residents with advanced dementia. JAMA 291(22):2734–2740, 2004 15187055

Mitchell SL, Teno JM, Kiely DK, et al: The clinical course of advanced dementia. N Engl J Med 361(16):1529–1538, 2009 19828530

Mitchell SL, Miller SC, Teno JM, et al: The Advanced Dementia Prognostic Tool: a risk score to estimate survival in nursing home residents with advanced dementia. J Pain Symptom Manage 40(5):639–651, 2010a 20621437

Mitchell SL, Miller SC, Teno JM, et al: Prediction of 6-month survival of nursing home residents with advanced dementia using ADEPT vs hospice eligibility guidelines. JAMA 304(17):1929–1935, 2010b 21045099

Mitchell SL, Black BS, Ersek M, et al: Advanced dementia: state of the art and priorities for the next decade. Ann Intern Med 156(1 Pt 1):45–51, 2012 22213494

Mohamed S, Rosenheck R, Lyketsos CG, et al: Caregiver burden in Alzheimer disease: cross-sectional and longitudinal patient correlates. Am J Geriatr Psychiatry 18(10):917–927, 2010 20808108

Mohamed S, Rosenheck R, Lyketsos CG, et al: Effect of second-generation antipsychotics on caregiver burden in Alzheimer's disease. J Clin Psychiatry 73(1):121–128, 2012 21939611

Nasreddine ZS, Phillips NA, Bédirian V, et al: The Montreal Cognitive Assessment, MoCA: a brief screening tool for mild cognitive impairment. Am J Geriatr Soc 53(4):695–699, 2005 15817019

National Hospice Organization: Medical guidelines for determining prognosis in selected non-cancer diseases. Hosp J 11(2):47–63, 1996 8949013

Passmore MJ: Neuropsychiatric symptoms of dementia: consent, quality of life, and dignity. Biomed Res Int 2013:230134, 2013 23853768

Porsteinsson AP, Drye LT, Pollock BG, et al; CitAD Research Group: Effect of citalopram on agitation in Alzheimer disease: the CitAD randomized clinical trial. JAMA 311(7):682–691, 2014 24549548

Reisberg B: Functional Assessment Staging (FAST). Psychopharmacol Bull 24(4):653–659, 1988 3249767

Rothenberg LR, Doberman D, Simon LE, et al: Patients surviving six months in hospice care: who are they? J Palliat Med 17(8):899–905, 2014 24933676

Sachs GA, Carter R, Holtz LR, et al: Cognitive impairment: an independent predictor of excess mortality: a cohort study. Ann Intern Med 155(5):300–308, 2011 21893623

Schneider LS, Dagerman KS, Insel P: Risk of death with atypical antipsychotic drug treatment for dementia: meta-analysis of randomized placebo-controlled trials. JAMA 294(15):1934–1943, 2005 16234500

Seitz DP, Adunuri N, Gill SS, et al: Antidepressants for agitation and psychosis in dementia. Cochrane Database Syst Rev (2):CD008191, 2011 21328305

Seitz DP, Brisbin S, Herrmann N, et al: Efficacy and feasibility of nonpharmacological interventions for neuropsychiatric symptoms of dementia in long term care: a systematic review. J Am Med Dir Assoc 13(6):503.e2–506.e2, 2012 22342481

Seitz DP, Gill SS, Herrmann N, et al: Pharmacological treatments for neuropsychiatric symptoms of dementia in long-term care: a systematic review. Int Psychogeriatr 25(2):185–203, 2013 23083438

Shega JW, Hougham GW, Stocking CB, et al: Patients dying with dementia: experience at the end of life and impact of hospice care. J Pain Symptom Manage 35(5):499–507, 2008 18261878

Shulman KI, Herrmann N, Brodaty H, et al: IPA survey of brief cognitive screening instruments. Int Psychogeriatr 18(2):281–294, 2006 16466586

Smith T, Gildeh N, Holmes C: The Montreal Cognitive Assessment: validity and utility in a memory clinic setting. Can J Psychiatry 52(5):329–332, 2007 17542384

Sokol EW: National plan to address Alzheimer's disease offers hope for new home care and hospice provisions. Caring 32(1):24–27, 2013 23634509

Steinberg M, Lyketsos CG: Atypical antipsychotic use in patients with dementia: managing safety concerns. Am J Psychiatry 169(9):900–906, 2012 22952071

Tejada-Vera B: Mortality from Alzheimer's disease in the United States: data for 2000 and 2010. NCHS Data Brief (116):1–8, 2013

Tjia J, Briesacher BA, Peterson D, et al: Use of medications of questionable benefit in advanced dementia. JAMA Intern Med 174(11):1763–1771, 2014 25201279

Torke AM, Holtz LR, Hui S, et al: Palliative care for patients with dementia: a national survey. J Am Geriatr Soc 58(11):2114–2121, 2010 21054292

Velayudhan L, Ryu SH, Raczek M, et al: Review of brief cognitive tests for patients with suspected dementia. Int Psychogeriatr 26(8):1247–1262, 2014 24685119

Vitaliano PP, Zhang J, Scanlan JM: Is caregiving hazardous to one's physical health? A meta-analysis. Psychol Bull 129(6):946–972, 2003 14599289

Wang J, Yu JT, Wang HF, et al: Pharmacological treatment of neuropsychiatric symptoms in Alzheimer's disease: a systematic review and meta-analysis. J Neurol Neurosurg Psychiatry 86(1):101–109, 2015 24876182

Wang PS, Schneeweiss S, Avorn J, et al: Risk of death in elderly users of conventional vs atypical antipsychotic medications. N Engl J Med 353(22):2335–2341, 2005 16319382

Wendler D, Rid A: Systematic review: the effect on surrogates of making treatment decisions for others. Ann Intern Med 154(5):336–346, 2011 21357911

Additional Resources

Alzheimer's Association. Web site at: http://www.alz.org.

Education in Palliative and End-of-Life-Care for Long-Term Care (EPEC-LTC). Available at: http://www.epec.net/epec_ltc.php?curid=4. Accessed July 25, 2015.

Hughes JC: How We Think About Dementia: Personhood, Rights, Ethics, the Arts and What They Mean for Care. London, Jessica Kingsley, 2014

Martin G, Sabbagh MN: Palliative Care for Advanced Alzheimer's and Dementia: Guidelines for Evidence-Based Care. New York, Springer, 2011

National Hospice and Palliative Care Organization: Caring for persons with Alzheimer's and other dementias: guidelines for hospice providers. National Hospice and Palliative Care Organization, 2007. Available at: http://www.nhpco.org/sites/default/files/public/Dementia-Caring-Guide-final.pdf. Accessed July 25, 2015.

Shega JW, Levine SK: UNIPAC 9: Caring for Patients With Chronic Illnesses: Dementia, COPD, and CHF. UNIPAC Self Study Program, 4th Edition. Edited by Storey CP Jr. Glenview, IL, American Academy of Hospice and Palliative Medicine, 2012. Available at: http://www.aahpm.org/resources/default/unipac-4th-edition.html. Accessed July 25, 2015.

Center to Advance Palliative Care, Fast Facts

Morrison LJ, Liao S: Fast Fact #174: Dementia medications in palliative care. Available at: https://www.capc.org/fast-facts/174-dementia-medications-palliative-care/. Accessed July 25, 2015.

Tsai S, Arnold RM: Fast Fact #150: Prognostication in dementia. Available at: https://www.capc.org/fast-facts/150-prognostication-dementia/. Accessed July 25, 2015.

7

Insomnia

Chapter Overview

This chapter reviews the approach to addressing insomnia, a common symptom in palliative care patients, which can significantly worsen quality of life. Broadly, assessment and management of insomnia mirror the approach used in healthy populations. Some important differences exist, however, including the contribution of disease-related factors and high levels of spiritual and existential distress, as well as the vulnerability to adverse effects of medication among patients with serious, life-threatening illness. Nonpharmacological approaches should always be optimized, with pharmacological interventions reserved for refractory cases and used in time-limited therapeutic trials. Despite being a common condition among palliative care patients, insomnia can often be effectively treated, thereby contributing to significant improvements in quality of life.

Sleep disturbances are common among patients with serious medical illness, with estimates ranging from approximately 30% to 70% of patients in palliative care settings (Mercadante et al. 2004). Insomnia is a particular problem among patients with cancer, in whom it often clusters with fatigue, depression,

149

and pain (Davis and Goforth 2014; Davis et al. 2014), as well as among hospitalized patients and those living in institutional settings such as nursing facilities. Insomnia has been shown to contribute significantly to poor quality of life in both general and palliative care populations, with negative impacts on cognition, social functioning, and both physical and mental health (Induru and Walsh 2014; Kvale and Shuster 2006; Naeim et al. 2014; Rodriguez et al. 2015). Of particular relevance to the psychiatrist, insomnia is frequently a symptom that can be quickly addressed, through either nonpharmacological approaches or drug treatments, thereby providing swift and meaningful symptom relief, and often enabling effective rapport with patients who might otherwise be reluctant to allow the psychiatrist's involvement.

Classification and Causes

Broadly, insomnia may involve problems with sleep initiation (difficulty falling asleep), sleep maintenance (difficulty staying asleep), premature awakening, difficulty experiencing restorative sleep, and/or daytime symptoms resulting from poor sleep such as fatigue or inattention. Both the *Diagnostic and Statistical Manual of Mental Disorders,* 5th Edition (DSM-5; American Psychiatric Association 2013), and the *International Classification of Sleep Disorders,* Third Edition (ICSD-3; American Academy of Sleep Medicine 2014), provide useful classification/diagnostic approaches to insomnia. In DSM-5, insomnia disorder and the residual category "other specified insomnia disorder" are most closely aligned with the kinds of sleep disturbance commonly encountered in palliative care settings; the criteria and description, respectively, of these diagnoses are provided in Tables 7–1 and 7–2. The ICSD-3 delineates sleep disturbances in terms of the duration of symptoms: "short-term insomnia" involves a sleep disturbance that has been present for less than 3 months and that has become a significant, independent source of distress, whereas "chronic insomnia" describes a sleep disturbance that has lasted 3 months or more and that is marked by frequent occurrence (at least three times per week), sleep latency, periods of nighttime wakefulness, or premature morning arousal. Sleep problems related to falling or staying asleep, but not fully meeting either of the other classifications, are referred to as "other insomnias" (American Academy of Sleep Medicine 2014).

Table 7–1. DSM-5 diagnostic criteria for insomnia disorder

A. A predominant complaint of dissatisfaction with sleep quantity or quality, associated with one (or more) of the following symptoms:

1. Difficulty initiating sleep. (In children, this may manifest as difficulty initiating sleep without caregiver intervention.)

2. Difficulty maintaining sleep, characterized by frequent awakenings or problems returning to sleep after awakenings. (In children, this may manifest as difficulty returning to sleep without caregiver intervention.)

3. Early-morning awakening with inability to return to sleep.

B. The sleep disturbance causes clinically significant distress or impairment in social, occupational, educational, academic, behavioral, or other important areas of functioning.

C. The sleep difficulty occurs at least 3 nights per week.

D. The sleep difficulty is present for at least 3 months.

E. The sleep difficulty occurs despite adequate opportunity for sleep.

F. The insomnia is not better explained by and does not occur exclusively during the course of another sleep-wake disorder (e.g., narcolepsy, a breathing-related sleep disorder, a circadian rhythm sleep-wake disorder, a parasomnia).

G. The insomnia is not attributable to the physiological effects of a substance (e.g., a drug of abuse, a medication).

H. Coexisting mental disorders and medical conditions do not adequately explain the predominant complaint of insomnia.

Specify if:
  With non–sleep disorder mental comorbidity, including substance use disorders
  With other medical comorbidity
  With other sleep disorder

Specify if:
  Episodic: Symptoms last at least 1 month but less than 3 months.
  Persistent: Symptoms last 3 months or longer.
  Recurrent: Two (or more) episodes within the space of 1 year.

Note: Acute and short-term insomnia (i.e., symptoms lasting less than 3 months but otherwise meeting all criteria with regard to frequency, intensity, distress, and/or impairment) should be coded as an other specified insomnia disorder.

Note. Criteria set above contains only the diagnostic criteria and specifiers; refer to DSM-5 for the full criteria set, including coding and reporting procedures.

Source. DSM-5 criteria for insomnia disorder reprinted from *Diagnostic and Statistical Manual of Mental Disorders,* 5th Edition. Washington, DC, American Psychiatric Association, 2013, pp. 362–363. Used with permission. Copyright © 2013 American Psychiatric Association.

Table 7–2.   DSM-5 other specified insomnia disorder

This category applies to presentations in which symptoms characteristic of insomnia disorder that cause clinically significant distress or impairment in social, occupational, or other important areas of functioning predominate but do not meet the full criteria for insomnia disorder or any of the disorders in the sleep-wake disorders diagnostic class. The other specified insomnia disorder category is used in situations in which the clinician chooses to communicate the specific reason that the presentation does not meet the criteria for insomnia disorder or any specific sleep-wake disorder. This is done by recording "other specified insomnia disorder" followed by the specific reason (e.g., "brief insomnia disorder").

Examples of presentations that can be specified using the "other specified" designation include the following:

1. **Brief insomnia disorder:** Duration is less than 3 months.

2. **Restricted to nonrestorative sleep:** Predominant complaint is nonrestorative sleep unaccompanied by other sleep symptoms such as difficulty falling asleep or remaining asleep.

Source.   DSM-5 category other specified insomnia disorder reprinted from *Diagnostic and Statistical Manual of Mental Disorders,* 5th Edition. Washington, DC, American Psychiatric Association, 2013, p. 420. Used with permission. Copyright © 2013 American Psychiatric Association.

In both classification systems, insomnias are often caused or precipitated by an external condition—such as an acute stressor, a change in medication, or an environmental factor—and in palliative care populations, such causes can be numerous. Table 7–3 lists some of the common causes of insomnia in palliative care settings. Accurate identification of an underlying cause is often key to the successful management of insomnia, because interventions vary substantially (e.g., although hypnotic medications are highly effective in treating some forms of insomnia, they are likely to worsen insomnia that results from delirium).

Assessment and Management

An overview of the approach to addressing insomnia in palliative care populations is provided in Figure 7–1. A comprehensive assessment, derived largely from the patient's self-report and knowledge of the patient's underlying medical disease, will help to guide interventions to address insomnia. As with

Table 7–3.   Common causes of insomnia in palliative care

Cause	Description
Delirium	Sleep disruption is a frequent sign of delirium, often marked by sleep-wake cycle disturbance or problems with sleep initiation or maintenance (LeGrand 2012).
Psychiatric conditions	*Mood disorders:* Insomnia is a common symptom associated with mood disorders such as major depression and bipolar disorder. Patients frequently experience negative ruminations, especially as they are attempting to quiet their mind to fall asleep. *Anxiety disorders:* Insomnia can occur with any of the anxiety disorders, especially those seen commonly in the palliative care population: panic disorder, generalized anxiety disorder, adjustment disorder with anxiety, and posttraumatic stress disorder (Mercadante et al. 2004; Morin and Benca 2012).
Medical conditions	Many medical conditions can contribute to or cause sleep disturbances. Conditions commonly encountered in palliative care settings include the following • Cancer (Savard et al. 2011) • Chronic obstructive pulmonary disease and other respiratory illnesses (Budhiraja et al. 2012) • Parkinson's disease, often associated with worsening of movements at night (Politis et al. 2010)
Pain	Pain can contribute to insomnia and can be worsened by sleep disturbance (Raymond et al. 2001).
Medication adverse effects	Many medications commonly used in palliative care settings can contribute to insomnia (Weinhouse 2008). Typical offenders include the following: • Opioids • Steroids • Stimulants • β-Receptor agonists • Some antidepressants

Table 7–3.   Common causes of insomnia in palliative
care *(continued)*

Cause	Description
Environmental	Environmental changes frequently cause or contribute to insomnia, particularly in the hospital or other institutional settings (Venkateshiah and Collop 2012). Examples include the following: • Alarms (intravenous pumps, bed alarms, monitoring devices, pagers, phones) • Patient care activities (physician and nursing assessments, medication administration, phlebotomy) • Unit activities and conversations • Lighting

other symptom management strategies in palliative care, effective treatment of insomnia begins with efforts to identify and address any physical or psychiatric conditions that may cause or contribute to the sleep disturbance. For example, factors such as pain, dyspnea, nausea, nocturnal urination, delirium, anxiety, or depression are often associated with poor sleep; improvement in those conditions very often leads to resolution of insomnia. Collateral information from the patient's sleep partner can be helpful as well. Unique to palliative care settings, spiritual and existential distress (and sometimes simply the fear of dying in one's sleep) can frequently be the cause of insomnia, and a careful exploration of this possibility—with assistance from a palliative care chaplain, for example—is sometimes necessary before any improvement in sleep can be achieved.

Beyond the initial approach of identifying and addressing underlying causes, nonpharmacological interventions and drug treatments also have an important role in the management of insomnia.

Nonpharmacological Interventions

Nonpharmacological interventions should always be employed. As described in Table 7–4, these may include environmental modifications, adjustment of medication, and a variety of behavioral and cognitive interventions. With regard to environmental changes, institutional settings and clinical practice

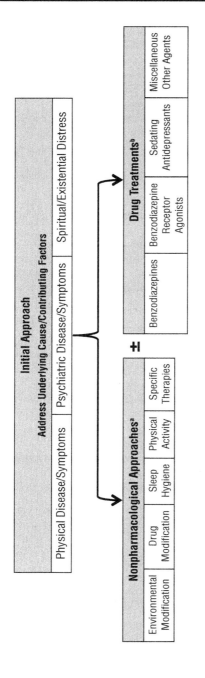

Figure 7–1.   Overview of approach to addressing insomnia in palliative care populations. [a]See Table 7–4 ("Nonpharmacological interventions for insomnia"). [b]See Table 7–5 ("Drug treatments for insomnia in palliative care").

Table 7–4.   Nonpharmacological interventions for insomnia

Intervention	Description
Environmental modification	Limit nighttime disruptions: • Avoid unnecessary sleeptime bedside care. • Minimize arousal when interventions are necessary (avoid overhead lights, reduce noise, etc.). Provide stimulating activity during the day. Provide exposure to natural light during the day. Minimize exposure to TV, computer screens, and so on, near bedtime.
Drug modification	Schedule routine medications after 6 A.M. and before 10 P.M. Avoid bedtime use of stimulating medication. Ensure that scheduled medications are not given more frequently than necessary (e.g., dexamethasone in the morning is preferred rather than four times daily).
Sleep hygiene	Limit consumption of caffeine (reduce overall consumption, and avoid consumption after 2 P.M.). Follow a consistent schedule for sleeping and waking. Develop and follow a consistent, relaxing routine prior to bedtime. Do not exercise or drink alcohol close to bedtime. Limit exposure to screens (TV, computer, tablet, smartphone, etc.) within ~30 minutes of bedtime. Reserve the bed for sleep or sex only: • Do not, for example, do work or watch TV in bed. • Do not remain in bed without sleeping; if unable to sleep after ~20 minutes, get out of bed and do something nonstimulating, then try again.
Physical activity	Light physical activity in the daytime can help promote restful sleep.
Specific therapies	Relaxation therapies Stimulus-control therapies Sleep restriction therapies Cognitive-behavioral therapy

patterns are rarely designed with the promotion of restful sleep in mind (Venkateshiah and Collop 2012). Hence, patients and care teams need to be proactive and deliberate about limiting nighttime disruptions. When possible, bedside care (vitals, labs, bathing, etc.) should not be scheduled during sleeptime, and any essential nighttime care should minimize arousal (e.g., by limiting noise and avoiding the use of overhead lights). Earplugs and eye masks may be helpful for some patients. In terms of medication adjustments, dosing times should be chosen to minimize sleep disruption (e.g., after 6 A.M. and before 10 P.M.). When clinically appropriate, stimulating agents should not be given after 2 P.M. Many agents with long half-lives (e.g., dexamethasone) are habitually scheduled in divided doses (three or four times daily), although it is often acceptable clinically to provide such medications once daily instead. Behavioral interventions to ameliorate sleep may include light physical activity (Montgomery and Dennis 2002) and assiduous attention to the elements of healthy sleep hygiene (see Table 7–4). Finally, data support the use of several specific therapies in the management of insomnia, including relaxation therapies, stimulus-control therapies, sleep restriction therapies, and cognitive-behavioral therapy (Davis and Goforth 2014; Garland et al. 2014; Induru and Walsh 2014; McCurry et al. 2007). Most data seem to support a combination of strategies as the most efficacious approach.

Pharmacological Interventions

In general, drug treatments should be reserved for cases in which the nonpharmacological strategies have been optimized yet insomnia persists. Table 7–5 provides details on pharmacological options for the management of insomnia. Benzodiazepines, benzodiazepine receptor agonists, sedating antidepressants, and agents from assorted other drug classes are among the options for drug treatment of insomnia in palliative care. Current data do not support the selection of one agent over another from the standpoint of efficacy; in practice, agents are chosen on the basis of side effects, familiarity, drug interactions, and other factors. Many experts recommend caution with the use of benzodiazepines and benzodiazepine receptor agonists in palliative care populations, in particular, due to the risk of adverse effects and falls (Davis and Goforth 2014; Kvale and Shuster 2006).

Table 7–5.   Drug treatments for insomnia in palliative care

Drug by class	Suggested dosing, titration	Notes
Benzodiazepines		
		Effective sedative-hypnotics, but use with caution in palliative care setting
		Cause sedation, confusion/delirium, falls, disinhibition
Lorazepam	0.25–2 mg PO qhs	Wide dose range; adjust to desired effect or side effect
		Onset: 30–120 min
		Half-life: 12–14 hrs
		Safer in liver failure than clonazepam
		Available routes: PO (tabs, liq), SL, SC, IM, IV
Temazepam	7.5 mg PO qhs	Onset: 30–60 min; in some patients may take up to 2 hrs
	Titrate to 15 or 30 mg PO qhs	Half-life: 8–15 hrs
		Safer in liver failure than clonazepam
		Available routes: PO (caps)
Benzodiazepine receptor agonists		
Eszopiclone	1–3 mg PO qhs	Dose conservatively in elderly and debilitated patients
		Onset: 30–60 min (high-fat foods delay absorption)
		Half-life: 6 hrs
		Adverse effects include sedation, dizziness, amnesia
		Studies up to 6 months did not show tolerance or dependence

Table 7–5. Drug treatments for insomnia in palliative care (*continued*)

Drug by class	Suggested dosing, titration	Notes
Benzodiazepine receptor agonists (*continued*)		
Zaleplon	5–10 mg PO qhs	Dose conservatively in elderly or those with low body weight or hepatic impairment Onset: 30 min (high-fat foods delay absorption) Half-life: 1 hr Adverse effects include sedation, dizziness, amnesia Available routes: PO (caps)
Zolpidem	5–10 mg PO qhs ER formulation: 6.25–12.5 mg PO qhs	Dose conservatively in women, elderly, low body weight Onset: 30–60 min Half-life: 3 hrs Adverse effects include sedation, dizziness, confusion, complex sleep behaviors, parasomnias Linked to increased falls in hospitalized elderly patients Available routes: PO (tabs)

Table 7–5.   Drug treatments for insomnia in palliative care (*continued*)

Drug by class	Suggested dosing, titration	Notes
Sedating antidepressants		
Trazodone	25–100 mg PO qhs	May repeat dose if ineffective after 1 hr; wide dose range; some patients require 400 mg qhs Onset: 1 hr Half-life: 7 hrs Adverse effects include sedation, dry mouth, priapism (rare) Does not interfere with normal sleep architecture Not associated with tolerance or dependence Available routes: PO (tabs)
Mirtazapine	7.5–15 mg PO qhs	Exact mechanism of action unknown (increases central serotonergic and noradrenergic activity) Half-life: 20–40 hrs Useful for insomnia at the lower end of the dose range; sedating effect decreases with titration Onset for insomnia usually occurs within a small number of days Adverse effects include orthostatic hypotension; also stimulates appetite Available routes: PO (tabs, ODT)

Table 7–5.   Drug treatments for insomnia in palliative care *(continued)*

Drug by class	Suggested dosing, titration	Notes
Sedating antidepressants *(continued)*		
Doxepin	10–50 mg PO qhs	Use lower doses in elderly and medically ill patients Onset: 30 min Half-life: 8–24 hrs At hypnotic doses, action is primarily related to blockade of histamine receptors Available routes: PO (tabs, caps, soln), TD (cream; highly variable absorption)
Amitriptyline, Imipramine	10–25 mg PO qhs Increase by 10–25 mg q 3–5 days Usual effective dose ~50–150 mg/day	TCAs Adverse effects include high anticholinergic load (increased risk of delirium), orthostatic hypotension, cardiotoxicity Many drug-drug interactions (TCAs are CYP2D6 substrates; combination with inhibitors will increase dose of TCA) Available routes: PO (tabs)

Table 7–5.   Drug treatments for insomnia in palliative care *(continued)*

Drug by class	Suggested dosing, titration	Notes
Miscellaneous other agents		
Ramelteon	8 mg PO qhs	A selective melatonin receptor agonist Very low bioavailability and variable absorption; may require significant escalation in dose to reach effect (up to 64 mg) Onset: 20–60 min Half-life: 2–5 hrs Adverse effects include sedation, dizziness, headache Significant drug-drug interactions along the CYP pathway Available routes: PO (tabs)
Suvorexant	10–20 mg PO qhs	An orexin receptor antagonist Onset: 30–60 min (delayed with food) Half-life: 12 hrs Adverse effects include headache, dizziness, sedation Do not use with strong CYP3A inhibitors Do not use in severe hepatic impairment Available routes: PO (tabs)

Table 7–5. Drug treatments for insomnia in palliative care *(continued)*

Drug by class	Suggested dosing, titration	Notes
Miscellaneous other agents (continued)		
Melatonin	2–10 mg PO qhs	Available OTC, not FDA regulated; potency may vary Adverse effects include headache, nightmares, dyspepsia Generally well tolerated; may be a low-risk agent for treatment of insomnia Check drug-drug interactions before prescribing Available routes: PO (tabs, caps, ODT, tea)
Diphenhydramine	12.5–50 mg PO qhs	Available OTC Onset: 30–120 min Half-life: 4–8 hrs Adverse effects are anticholinergic (high risk of delirium in medically ill populations) Available routes: PO (tabs, caps, elixir), IM, IV

Note. Dosing guidelines reflect a general initial strategy based on the clinical experience of the authors and current drug references (Micromedex DRUGDEX 2014). Local experts and other resources should be consulted for specific concerns (e.g., dosing strategies in incomplete responders, or dose adjustments in hepatic/renal insufficiency). Users should consult with current references for FDA-labeled indications. caps=capsules; CYP=cytochrome P450; ER=extended release; FDA=U.S. Food and Drug Administration; IM=intramuscular; IV=intravenous; liq=liquid; ODT=orally disintegrating tablet; OTC=over the counter; PO=per oral; qhs=at bedtime; SC=subcutaneous; SL=sublingual; soln=solution; tabs=tablets; TCA=tricyclic antidepressant; TD=transdermal.

Depending on the stage and type of illness, palliative care patients are often at heightened risk for experiencing adverse effects from typical sleep aids. For this reason, careful drug selection and monitoring are critical. In addition, it is not uncommon for patients who have historically used a sleep aid without adverse effects to develop new complications in the context of an advancing medical disease. For example, an elderly patient who has historically used zolpidem safely may become increasingly at risk for falls or delirium in the setting of progression of an underlying medical disease (Kolla et al. 2013). Hence, drug treatment strategies should include 1) selecting agents with the least likelihood of causing adverse effects, 2) using the lowest effective therapeutic dose, and 3) ongoing monitoring for clinical improvement and side effects, especially as the patient's condition changes.

Conclusions and Key Points

- Insomnia is common among patients in palliative care settings, and it contributes to poor quality of life.

- Medical and psychiatric conditions can cause or exacerbate insomnia in palliative care settings, as can spiritual or existential distress.

- Addressing underlying conditions should be a first step in treating insomnia.

- Environmental and behavioral interventions should always be optimized.

- Drug treatments should be used cautiously in patients with advanced illness to avoid potential adverse effects.

- Evidence does not support the preferential use of any particular drug treatment.

- Pharmacological interventions should be frequently reassessed as the patient's condition changes to ensure that they remain safe and effective.

References

American Academy of Sleep Medicine: International Classification of Sleep Disorders, 3rd Edition. Darien, IL, American Academy of Sleep Medicine, 2014

American Psychiatric Association: Diagnostic and Statistical Manual of Mental Disorders, 5th Edition. Arlington, VA, American Psychiatric Association, 2013

Budhiraja R, Parthasarathy S, Budhiraja P, et al: Insomnia in patients with COPD. Sleep 35(3):369–375, 2012 22379243

Davis MP, Goforth H: Fighting insomnia and battling lethargy: the yin and yang of palliative care. Curr Oncol Rep 16(4):377, 2014 24535303

Davis MP, Khoshknabi D, Walsh D, et al: Insomnia in patients with advanced cancer. Am J Hosp Palliat Care 31(4):365–373, 2014 23616275

Garland SN, Johnson JA, Savard J, et al: Sleeping well with cancer: a systematic review of cognitive behavioral therapy for insomnia in cancer patients. Neuropsychiatr Dis Treat 10:1113–1124, 2014 24971014

Induru RR, Walsh D: Cancer-related insomnia. Am J Hosp Palliat Care 31(7):777–785, 2014 24142594

Kolla BP, Lovely JK, Mansukhani MP, et al: Zolpidem is independently associated with increased risk of inpatient falls. J Hosp Med 8(1):1–6, 2013 23165956

Kvale EA, Shuster JL: Sleep disturbance in supportive care of cancer: a review. J Palliat Med 9(2):437–450, 2006 16629573

LeGrand SB: Delirium in palliative medicine: a review. J Pain Symptom Manage 44(4): 583–594, 2012 22682074

McCurry SM, Logsdon RG, Teri L, et al: Evidence-based psychological treatments for insomnia in older adults. Psychol Aging 22(1):18–27, 2007 17385979

Mercadante S, Girelli D, Casuccio A: Sleep disorders in advanced cancer patients: prevalence and factors associated. Support Care Cancer 12(5):355–359, 2004 15064937

Micromedex DRUGDEX (Internet database). Ann Arbor, MI, Truven Health Analytics, 2014. Available at: www.micromedexsolutions.com. Subscription required to view.

Montgomery P, Dennis J: Physical exercise for sleep problems in adults aged 60+. Cochrane Database Syst Rev (4):CD003404, 2002 12519595

Morin CM, Benca R: Chronic insomnia. Lancet 379(9821):1129–1141, 2012 22265700

Naeim A, Aapro M, Subbarao R, et al: Supportive care considerations for older adults with cancer. J Clin Oncol 32(24):2627–2634, 2014 25071112

Politis M, Wu K, Molloy S, et al: Parkinson's disease symptoms: the patient's perspective. Mov Disord 25(11):1646–1651, 2010 20629164

Raymond I, Nielsen TA, Lavigne G, et al: Quality of sleep and its daily relationship to pain intensity in hospitalized adult burn patients. Pain 92(3):381–388, 2001 11376911

Rodriguez JC, Dzierzewski JM, Alessi CA: Sleep problems in the elderly. Med Clin North Am 99(2):431–439, 2015 25700593

Savard J, Ivers H, Villa J, et al: Natural course of insomnia comorbid with cancer: an 18-month longitudinal study. J Clin Oncol 29(26):3580–3586, 2011 21825267

Venkateshiah SB, Collop NA: Sleep and sleep disorders in the hospital. Chest 141(5): 1337–1345, 2012 22553268

Weinhouse GL: Pharmacology I: effects on sleep of commonly used ICU medications. Crit Care Clin 24(3):477–491, vi, 2008 18538196

Additional Resources

Education in Palliative and End-of-Life-Care for Oncology (EPEC-Oncology). Module 3l: Insomnia. Available at: http://www.cancer.gov/cancertopics/cancerlibrary/epeco. Accessed July 27, 2015.

Center to Advance Palliative Care, Fast Facts

Arnold RM, Miller M, Mehta RS: Fast Fact #101: Insomnia: patient assessment. Available at: https://www.capc.org/fast-facts/101-insomnia-patient-assessment/. Accessed July 27, 2015.

Arnold RM, Miller M, Mehta RS: Fast Fact #104: Insomnia: non-pharmacologic treatments. Available at: https://www.capc.org/fast-facts/104-insomnia-non-pharmacologic-treatments/. Accessed July 27, 2015.

Arnold RM, Miller M, Mehta RS: Fast Fact #105: Insomnia: drug therapies. Available at: https://www.capc.org/fast-facts/105-insomnia-drug-therapies/. Accessed July 27, 2015.

8

Substance Use Disorders

This chapter provides an overview of the approach to identifying, managing, and mitigating the effects of substance use disorders in the palliative care setting. Because of the significant harms associated with problematic substance use—for the patient and family in particular, but also for clinicians and for society at large—expert, interdisciplinary care is essential to the successful management of palliative care patients with substance use problems. Problematic substance use should be targeted specifically, as an element of a comprehensive plan of care, because it can cause significant distress, can undermine disease- and symptom-directed therapies, and can limit the patient's success in accomplishing important developmental tasks near the end of life. Even for patients with a limited prognosis, such efforts can often help to alleviate suffering related to substance use disorders in the palliative care setting.

In the general population, as well as in palliative care populations, substance use disorders can cause immense suffering for the patient, family members, and frequently the providers caring for them. Although substance use disorders rarely develop de novo in the setting of treating acute cancer pain or other symptom management near the end of life, in the management of chronic noncancer pain, opioid therapy can lead to the development of a substance use disorder. Moreover, in both settings, long-standing substance use problems can present significant obstacles to the management of an advanced, serious medical illness (Ballantyne 2013).

Psychiatric expertise is often an essential component in the care of such patients. Anxiety disorders and mood disturbances are commonly comorbid with substance use disorders, for example, and management of anxiety and mood disorders is sometimes essential to alleviating distress that contributes to problematic substance use. Patients with substance use disorders often experience heightened psychosocial challenges (e.g., fractured relationships, inconsistent social support), which can limit the impact of interventions that hinge on mobilization of support. Countertransference issues can predominate as well, sometimes rooted in moral judgments and/or misinformed ideas about the etiology of substance use problems. Similarly, clinicians and family can mistakenly assume that addressing substance use problems in the palliative care setting is wasted effort, or that unlimited access to substances is a harm-free intervention and appropriate when time is short (Passik and Theobald 2000). These attitudes often result from a failure to appreciate that substance use disorders are rooted in a loss of control, and that efforts to restore control can help to alleviate suffering—even in individuals with a limited prognosis.

Epidemiology and Consequences

Substance use disorders are common in the United States, occurring in approximately 8.5% of individuals ages 12 years and older, and rates in men are roughly double those observed in women (Substance Abuse and Mental Health Services Administration 2013). In terms of specific conditions, alcohol use disorder occurs in approximately 18 million adults in the United States, where the 12-month prevalence is about 6.8% among individuals ages 12 years and older (Substance Abuse and Mental Health Services Administration 2013). Particularly relevant to treatment in the palliative care setting, opioid use disorders are common and increasing among adults in the United States. In 2013, more than 2 million individuals ages 12 years and older had an opioid use disorder, with roughly 75% of those cases related to prescription opioids (0.8% 12-month prevalence) and 25% related to heroin (0.2% 12-month prevalence) (Substance Abuse and Mental Health Services Administration 2015).

Substance use disorders are associated with major social, legal, and economic consequences in the general population. As a result, opioid prescribing has important ramifications for public health and policy. Perhaps most alarming, the increase in prescription drug misuse has closely paralleled a marked increase in deaths from prescription drug overdose: since 1999, deaths from opioid overdose have increased 265% among men and 400% among women (Substance Abuse and Mental Health Services Administration 2015). Such data bring into sharp relief the need for careful prescribing and risk management strategies, particularly among individuals with an existing substance use problem and a comorbid advanced medical illness.

Among patients receiving palliative care, there is little meaningful epidemiological data regarding the prevalence of specific substance use disorders. In a small series of ambulatory cancer patients who underwent a structured clinical interview, 5% met criteria for a substance use disorder (Derogatis et al. 1983). Many of the standard symptom management strategies in palliative care rely on aggressive use of controlled substances, including opioids, benzodiazepines, and even psychostimulants, each of which can be associated with problematic use. In the palliative care setting, it can be difficult to discern legitimate, controlled medical use from illegitimate, uncontrolled misuse—particularly when there is a prior history of misuse and/or an evolving pattern of physical symptoms due to the progression of disease.

Definitions

Psychiatric nomenclature for substance use disorders changed in 2013 with the release of the *Diagnostic and Statistical Manual of Mental Disorders,* 5th Edition (DSM-5; American Psychiatric Association 2013). Previously, distinctions were made between substance abuse and substance dependence, but now those concepts are unified under the single heading of "substance use disorder." Disorders are distinguished by the particular substance in question (e.g., opioid use disorder, alcohol use disorder). In addition, disorders are further specified by severity (mild, moderate, or severe, based on the number of symptoms present) and by the presence or absence of remission (early or sustained). Thus, the term *substance use disorder* can capture a wide range of behaviors, from those causing only mild problems to those resulting in serious and severe consequences. Of particular relevance to the palliative care setting, DSM-5 also specifically indicates that a substance use disorder should not be diagnosed when use occurs solely under appropriate medical supervision, even when tolerance or withdrawal arises (American Psychiatric Association 2013).

Table 8–1 provides DSM-5 criteria sets for opioid use disorder and alcohol use disorder, two conditions that are commonly seen in palliative care settings. Conceptually, the central, shared feature of all substance use disorders is the *loss of control* over the use of the substance, and symptoms can be usefully clustered in groupings related to impaired control, social consequences, dangerous use, and pharmacological phenomena (American Psychiatric Association 2013). By design, DSM-5 eschews the term *addiction* because of its imprecision and potentially negative connotations. Passik and Kirsh (2006) capture this more sharply: "the terms 'addiction' and 'addict' are particularly troublesome and often inappropriately applied to describe both aberrant drug use and phenomena related to tolerance or physical dependence. Clinicians and patients may use the word 'addicted' to describe compulsive drug taking in one patient and nothing more than the possibility for withdrawal in another" (p. 518). Consistent use of language helps to ensure that care is focused and specific, which is particularly important in the realm of substance use disorders, because lay terminology can often be laced with social or moral meanings (intended and unintended). Table 8–2 provides definitions for some terms commonly used in connection with substance use disorders.

Challenges in Diagnosis

When problematic substance use behaviors arise, careful consideration of a full differential diagnosis is critically important. In a patient with a serious physical illness receiving prescribed medication with high potential for misuse, it can be difficult to identify a substance use disorder. Similarly, in a patient with a known premorbid substance use disorder, it can be challenging to interpret substance-related behaviors in the context of a progressing serious illness. For example, the application of diagnostic criteria for opioid use disorder can be difficult when the escalation of opioids may serve a legitimate and essential medical purpose. In this setting, separate from particular diag-

Table 8–1.   DSM-5 criteria for alcohol use disorder and opioid use disorder

DSM-5 criteria for alcohol use disorder	DSM-5 criteria for opioid use disorder
A. A problematic pattern of alcohol use leading to clinically significant impairment or distress, as manifested by at least two of the following, occurring within a 12-month period:	A. A problematic pattern of opioid use leading to clinically significant impairment or distress, as manifested by at least two of the following, occurring within a 12-month period:
1. Alcohol is often taken in larger amounts or over a longer period than was intended.	1. Opioids are often taken in larger amounts or over a longer period than was intended.
2. There is a persistent desire or unsuccessful efforts to cut down or control alcohol use.	2. There is a persistent desire or unsuccessful efforts to cut down or control opioid use.
3. A great deal of time is spent in activities necessary to obtain alcohol, use alcohol, or recover from its effects.	3. A great deal of time is spent in activities necessary to obtain the opioid, use the opioid, or recover from its effects.
4. Craving, or a strong desire or urge to use alcohol.	4. Craving, or a strong desire or urge to use opioids.
5. Recurrent alcohol use resulting in a failure to fulfill major role obligations at work, school, or home.	5. Recurrent opioid use resulting in a failure to fulfill major role obligations at work, school, or home.
6. Continued alcohol use despite having persistent or recurrent social or interpersonal problems caused or exacerbated by the effects of alcohol.	6. Continued opioid use despite having persistent or recurrent social or interpersonal problems caused or exacerbated by the effects of opioids.
7. Important social, occupational, or recreational activities are given up or reduced because of alcohol use.	7. Important social, occupational, or recreational activities are given up or reduced because of opioid use.
8. Recurrent alcohol use in situations in which it is physically hazardous.	8. Recurrent opioid use in situations in which it is physically hazardous.

Table 8–1.   DSM-5 criteria for alcohol use disorder and opioid use disorder *(continued)*

DSM-5 criteria for alcohol use disorder *(cont'd)*	DSM-5 criteria for opioid use disorder *(cont'd)*
9. Alcohol use is continued despite knowledge of having a persistent or recurrent physical or psychological problem that is likely to have been caused or exacerbated by alcohol.	9. Continued opioid use despite knowledge of having a persistent or recurrent physical or psychological problem that is likely to have been caused or exacerbated by the substance.
10. Tolerance, as defined by either of the following:	10. Tolerance, as defined by either of the following:
a. A need for markedly increased amounts of alcohol to achieve intoxication or desired effect.	a. A need for markedly increased amounts of opioids to achieve intoxication or desired effect.
b. A markedly diminished effect with continued use of the same amount of alcohol.	b. A markedly diminished effect with continued use of the same amount of an opioid.
	Note: This criterion is not considered to be met for those taking opioids solely under appropriate medical supervision.
11. Withdrawal, as manifested by either of the following:	11. Withdrawal, as manifested by either of the following:
a. The characteristic withdrawal syndrome for alcohol (refer to Criteria A and B of the criteria set for alcohol withdrawal, pp. 499–500).	a. The characteristic opioid withdrawal syndrome (refer to Criteria A and B of the criteria set for opioid withdrawal, pp. 259–260).
b. Alcohol (or a closely related substance, such as a benzodiazepine) is taken to relieve or avoid withdrawal symptoms.	b. Opioids (or a closely related substance) are taken to relieve or avoid withdrawal symptoms.
	Note: This criterion is not considered to be met for those taking opioids solely under appropriate medical supervision.

Table 8–1.   DSM-5 criteria for alcohol use disorder and opioid use disorder (*continued*)

DSM-5 criteria for alcohol use disorder (*cont'd*)	DSM-5 criteria for opioid use disorder (*cont'd*)
Specify if:	*Specify* if:
In early remission: After full criteria for alcohol use disorder were previously met, none of the criteria for alcohol use disorder have been met for at least 3 months but for less than 12 months (with the exception that Criterion A4, "Craving, or a strong desire or urge to use alcohol," may be met).	**In early remission:** After full criteria for opioid use disorder were previously met, none of the criteria for opioid use disorder have been met for at least 3 months but for less than 12 months (with the exception that Criterion A4, "Craving, or a strong desire or urge to use opioids," may be met).
In sustained remission: After full criteria for alcohol use disorder were previously met, none of the criteria for alcohol use disorder have been met at any time during a period of 12 months or longer (with the exception that Criterion A4, "Craving, or a strong desire or urge to use alcohol," may be met).	**In sustained remission:** After full criteria for opioid use disorder were previously met, none of the criteria for opioid use disorder have been met at any time during a period of 12 months or longer (with the exception that Criterion A4, "Craving, or a strong desire or urge to use opioids," may be met).
Specify if:	*Specify* if:
In a controlled environment: This additional specifier is used if the individual is in an environment where access to alcohol is restricted.	**On maintenance therapy:** This additional specifier is used if the individual is taking a prescribed agonist medication such as methadone or buprenorphine and none of the criteria for opioid use disorder have been met for that class of medication (except tolerance to, or withdrawal from, the agonist). This category also applies to those individuals being maintained on a partial agonist, an agonist/antagonist, or a full antagonist such as oral naltrexone or depot naltrexone.
	In a controlled environment: This additional specifier is used if the individual is in an environment where access to opioids is restricted.

Table 8–1. DSM-5 criteria for alcohol use disorder and opioid use disorder *(continued)*

DSM-5 criteria for alcohol use disorder *(cont'd)*	DSM-5 criteria for opioid use disorder *(cont'd)*
Specify current severity:	*Specify* current severity:
Mild: Presence of 2–3 symptoms.	**Mild:** Presence of 2–3 symptoms.
Moderate: Presence of 4–5 symptoms.	**Moderate:** Presence of 4–5 symptoms.
Severe: Presence of 6 or more symptoms.	**Severe:** Presence of 6 or more symptoms.

Note. Criteria set above contains only the diagnostic criteria and specifiers; refer to DSM-5 for the full criteria set, including coding and reporting procedures.

Source. DSM-5 criteria for alcohol and opioid use disorder reprinted from *Diagnostic and Statistical Manual of Mental Disorders*, 5th Edition. Washington, DC, American Psychiatric Association, 2013, pp. 490–491 and 541–542. Used with permission. Copyright © 2013 American Psychiatric Association.

Table 8–2. Definitions of selected terms commonly used in association with substance use disorders

Substance use disorder	This is the current, preferred term for a psychiatric condition resulting from disordered use of substances. "The essential feature of a substance use disorder is a cluster of cognitive, behavioral, and physiological symptoms indicating that the individual continues using the substance despite significant substance-related problems" (American Psychiatric Association 2013, p. 483).
Substance abuse Substance dependence	Used in earlier versions of the *Diagnostic and Statistical Manual of Mental Disorders*, these diagnoses have been replaced by the term *substance use disorders*.
Addiction	"Addiction is a primary, chronic disease of brain reward, motivation, memory and related circuitry. Dysfunction in these circuits leads to characteristic biological, psychological, social and spiritual manifestations. This is reflected in an individual pathologically pursuing reward and/or relief by substance use and other behaviors. Addiction is characterized by inability to consistently abstain, impairment in behavioral control, craving, diminished recognition of significant problems with one's behaviors and interpersonal relationships, and a dysfunctional emotional response. Like other chronic diseases, addiction often involves cycles of relapse and remission. Without treatment or engagement in recovery activities, addiction is progressive and can result in disability or premature death" (American Society of Addiction Medicine 2011). Clinicians often use the term *addiction* interchangeably with *substance use disorder*. However, among the lay public (and even among clinicians at times), *addiction* can have other associated meanings, including those associated with moral judgments and character traits, which may be unintended or intended. Because of this imprecision in meaning, the term should be avoided in clinical settings.

Table 8–2. Definitions of selected terms commonly used in association with substance use disorders (*continued*)

Pseudoaddiction	Pseudoaddiction is an iatrogenic syndrome resulting from inadequate pain management, marked by escalation of behaviors aimed at obtaining effective pain relief, and often culminating in a crisis of mistrust between the patient and providers. It is distinguished from addiction in that symptoms resolve when effective pain relief is provided (Weissman and Haddox 1989).
Tolerance	"Tolerance is a state of adaptation in which exposure to a drug induces changes that result in a diminution of one or more of the drug's effects over time" (American Society of Addiction Medicine 2001). Tolerance may occur as part of a substance use disorder, or during appropriate, medically supervised use of a substance. Tolerance to the analgesic effects of opioids is generally believed to be rare.
Dependence	"Physical dependence is a state of adaptation that is manifested by a drug class specific withdrawal syndrome that can be produced by abrupt cessation, rapid dose reduction, decreasing blood level of the drug, and/or administration of an antagonist" (American Society of Addiction Medicine 2001). As with tolerance, dependence may occur as part of a substance use disorder, or during appropriate, medically supervised use of a substance.

nostic criteria, the conceptual framework of "loss of control" can often be helpful in identifying whether or not substance-related behaviors are problematic. Does the patient, for example, describe a sense of having lost control over the use of the prescribed medication? If the patient has experienced problems meeting role obligations (e.g., in relationships or at work), do these problems result from the medical disease or from uncontrolled use of a substance? Does the patient use the drug to achieve an intended therapeutic outcome (e.g., analgesia with opioids), or does use continue even after the therapeutic goal is achieved? These kinds of questions can help identify issues of loss of control in patients with comorbid substance use problems and serious medical disease.

Several other concepts can help to characterize and interpret substance-related behaviors in palliative care patients: aberrant drug use behaviors, pseudoaddiction, comorbid psychiatric illness, and pharmacokinetic variability.

Aberrant Drug Use Behaviors

Aberrant drug use behaviors encompass all patient behaviors outside normal medication adherence, ranging from potentially benign acts such as small, self-directed increases in the prescribed dose of an opioid, to egregious (or criminal) behaviors such as street sales of medication or forging prescriptions (Passik and Kirsh 2008). Table 8–3 provides a list of aberrant substance use behaviors. Among individuals with chronic pain, approximately 10%–15% exhibit aberrant drug behaviors, and risk factors appear to include a prior personal or family history of substance abuse, a history of drug-related legal problems, a history of mental illness, younger age, and male sex. Depression, severity of pain, income, and education do not appear to be risk factors (Ives et al. 2006; Michna et al. 2004).

Pseudoaddiction

Aberrant behaviors may or may not indicate the presence of a substance use disorder. In fact, patients with inadequately treated pain often will act in ways that mimic substance use behaviors. Pseudoaddiction, described in Table 8–2, is an iatrogenic condition marked by aberrant drug use behavior that results

Table 8–3.   Aberrant substance use behaviors

Mildly aberrant behaviors

    Requests for specific pain medications

    Aggressive complaints about the need for medication

    Using drugs prescribed for a friend or family member

    Frequent prescription losses

    Hoarding drugs

    Occasional unsanctioned dose escalation

Highly aberrant behaviors

    Forging prescriptions

    Obtaining drugs from nonmedical sources (e.g., stealing from others)

    Sale of prescription drugs

    Altering the route or drug delivery system (e.g., crushing sustained-release tablets for snorting or injecting)

Source.   Adapted from Passik et al. 2002.

from unrelieved pain (Weissman and Haddox 1989). Importantly, effective pain relief extinguishes aberrant behaviors that result from pseudoaddiction (a feature that distinguishes pseudoaddiction from a substance use disorder). Of course, in patients with a known substance use disorder and a legitimate clinical need for medication with a high potential for abuse, both pseudoaddiction and disordered substance use can co-occur. Furthermore, the significance of pseudoaddiction in the setting of noncancer chronic pain has been reevaluated, given the role it may have played in providing justification for escalating opioid doses—a strategy that increasingly appears to provide limited benefit and substantial risk of harm (Passik et al. 2011).

Comorbid Psychiatric Illness

Psychiatric illnesses such as anxiety disorders, affective disturbances, and personality disorders are highly comorbid with substance use disorders. According to findings from the National Survey on Drug Use and Health, 8.4 million adults in 2012 had both a diagnosed non-substance-related mental illness and a substance use disorder (Substance Abuse and Mental Health Services Administration 2013). Other mental illnesses may influence substance use disorders in a variety of ways. For example, serious character pathology can underlie aberrant drug behaviors entirely, and untreated disturbances of anxiety or mood may amplify somatic experiences (and perceived need for symptom-driven interventions) or produce distress that contributes to substance use (Kirsh and Passik 2006). Hence, careful identification of comorbid psychiatric conditions can help in contextualizing and interpreting aberrant behaviors, and effective management of comorbid psychiatric illness is an essential complement to comprehensive care planning for patients with substance use disorders.

Pharmacogenetic Variability

Recent studies have revealed a high degree of pharmacogenetic variability in metabolic enzymatic pathways, which may contribute to variability in patients' responses to opioid medications. Depending on the pace and completeness of drug metabolism, patients may experience a lack of therapeutic effect, shortened duration of effect, or increased adverse effects, relative to expected norms (Kirsh et al. 2014). For example, an ultrarapid metabolizer may seek (and need) more frequent dosing than a drug's typical half-life would predict. Therefore, when a patient does not respond as expected to a particular agent, it is important to consider the possibility of metabolic variability among the potential causes. In such cases, there may be a role for pharmacogenetic testing to help interpret atypical drug responses (de Leon et al. 2006).

Clinical Management

Effective clinical management of substance use disorders in the palliative care setting generally requires the coordination of multiple approaches aimed at ensuring adequate symptom relief, creating opportunities for restoration of control (for the patient, family, and clinicians), minimizing harm from continued problematic substance use, and promoting continued growth and development as life comes to a close. Passik and Weinreb (2000) have recommended a useful general approach, organized around "the 4 A's": ensuring adequate *analgesia,* focusing on *activities* of daily living, responding to *adverse* events, and monitoring for *aberrant* behaviors. "The 4 A's reflect a therapy that offers pain relief that makes a true difference in the patient's life, stabilizes or improves psychosocial functioning, manages side effects, does not compromise important areas of functioning, and provides an intact mechanism to assess and control aberrant behaviors" (Passik and Kirsh 2005, p. 84). Table 8–4 describes some of the basic elements of the management of substance use disorders in palliative care.

Risk Stratification and Management

Assessing and characterizing aberrant behaviors, before and during treatment, can be useful in risk stratification and in developing strategies for safe medication therapy. Aberrant behaviors alone do not signify the presence of a substance use disorder; instead, they signal a need for close attention, further exploration, and careful care planning. Repeated observations over time, careful psychiatric assessment, and close monitoring can all be appropriate responses when aberrant behaviors arise or escalate. The seriousness of aberrant behavior should be considered carefully in determining risk stratification and appropriate responses. Less serious behaviors (e.g., occasional dose escalations) may be indicative of inadequately treated symptoms, whereas highly aberrant behaviors (e.g., drug diversion) are often more clearly related to a substance use disorder. Differentiating highly aberrant behaviors from mild behaviors assists the clinician in determining the most appropriate therapeutic intervention.

Screening Tools

Many experts recommend the systematic use of screening instruments, both before initiation of therapy and as a strategy for ongoing monitoring, to help identify patients at higher risk for problematic substance use and to detect the emergence of problematic behaviors during therapy (Smith et al. 2009; Wu et al. 2006). Tools that can be helpful in risk stratification include the following:

- The CAGE-AID (Cut down, Annoyed, Guilty, Eye-opener—Adapted to Include Drugs) is a 4-item instrument that allows for conjoint screening for misuse of alcohol and other drugs (Brown and Rounds 1995).

Table 8–4.   Management of substance use disorders in palliative care

Screening, risk stratification	Screen all patients prior to prescribing opioids and benzodiazepines for risk of current or future development of substance use disorders. Consider use of screening instruments such as the following: • CAGE-AID (Cut down, Annoyed, Guilty, Eye-opener—Adapted to Include Drugs; Brown and Rounds 1995) • Opioid Risk Tool (Barclay et al. 2014) • Screener and Opioid Assessment for Patients with Pain—Short Form (Koyyalagunta et al. 2013)
Differential diagnosis	Rule out pseudoaddiction. Rule out or treat comorbid psychiatric conditions (e.g., anxiety disorders, depression, personality disorders). Rule out delirium and dementia. Rule out pharmacogenetic variances.
Interdisciplinary team	Include professionals from various specialties: • Palliative care specialists (e.g., physician, nurse practitioner, social work, chaplain, pharmacist) • Mental health specialists with expertise in treating substance use disorders (e.g., psychiatrist, psychologist, social worker) Coordinate with substance use treatment programs when indicated. Coordinate with 12-step programs (e.g., a patient's sponsor).
Urine drug screening	Obtain random urine drug screens to help maintain honest communication about drug use and provide information about adherence and effectiveness of the treatment plan. Discuss positive results openly and without shame to facilitate the development and delivery of effective care.

Table 8–4.   Management of substance use disorders in palliative care *(continued)*

Prescriptions	When a substance use disorder has been diagnosed and opioids or benzodiazepines are needed, consider these guidelines: • Weekly refills; no early refills without clinic visit • Consistent use of prescription monitoring program data • Pill and patch counts at clinic visits • Use of patches or tamper-resistant, long-acting formulations • Avoidance of immediate-release formulations • Avoidance of intravenous route; if needed, use of piggy-back technique and slow infusions Increase rigidity of prescribing practices depending on severity of substance use disorder and aberrant behaviors. Consider higher dosages for patients with a history of opioid, benzodiazepine, or alcohol use disorders. "Prescribe" engagement in psychotherapy, nonpharmacological symptom management techniques, and 12-step programs when indicated.
Monitoring results	Ensure continued satisfactory symptom relief. Monitor overall quality of life, with treatment goal of improving quality. Assess for adverse effects of drug therapies; treat these aggressively. Remain vigilant for aberrant drug use behaviors.
Withdrawal	Manage symptoms aggressively, based on goals of care, overall disease state, and prognosis. Be vigilant for symptoms of withdrawal in all patients with disease progression and during acute inpatient admissions.
Harm reduction	Remember that complete abstinence may not be a realistic goal for some patients. Keep in mind that open communication and realistic goals may help the patient adhere to an effective treatment plan. Recall that the goal is to help the patient adhere to palliative and disease-directed therapies.

- The Opioid Risk Tool is a 5-item instrument that has been found to reliably predict the risk of developing aberrant substance use behaviors with opioid therapy for both chronic and cancer pain (Barclay et al. 2014; Ma et al. 2014).
- The Screener and Opioid Assessment for Patients with Pain—Short Form has been shown to have success, in inpatient and outpatient palliative care settings, in identifying patients at risk for substance use disorders (Childers et al. 2015; Koyyalagunta et al. 2013).

Of note, in the setting of chronic noncancer pain, there are mixed data supporting the effectiveness of these instruments in predicting aberrant drug behavior before initiation of therapy or in identifying such behavior after initiation of therapy (Chou et al. 2009).

Interdisciplinary Team

Reliance on a fully staffed interdisciplinary team is doubly important when trying to negotiate the challenges involved in treating patients in palliative care with comorbid substance use disorders. The team not only allows for necessary specialist care but also helps to buffer against the common experience of developing anger and frustration among providers caring for this challenging population. Team members often include the usual palliative care specialists, as well as mental health providers with experience or specific training in the treatment of substance use disorders. Management of the substance use disorder, depending on its stage and severity, often exceeds the scope of a typical palliative care team, and the mental health specialist can be helpful in providing coordination with substance use treatment programs. For patients participating in 12-step programs, the involvement of a sponsor in the palliative plan of care may help to mitigate the prohibitions these programs sometimes have against the use of any substance of abuse.

Ensuring frequent communication between care providers, through clinical rounds or other standardized formats, should be a regular part of caring for palliative care patients with substance use disorders. Such discussions should involve an ongoing clarification of treatment goals, review of adherence to the plan of care, revision of the plan of care when necessary, and overall coordination of care. This is especially important when multiple providers are involved in the patient's care.

Psychiatric Assessment

Because of the high comorbidity of substance use problems and other psychiatric illness, careful psychiatric assessment and treatment are often essential components of successful management of substance use disorders in palliative care. Kirsh and Passik (2006) noted that

> perceptive psychiatric assessment is crucial and may require evaluation by consultants who can elucidate the complex interactions among personality factors, non addiction-related psychiatric illness, addiction, and abuse. Some patients may be self-medicating symptoms of anxiety or depression insomnia, or problems of adjustment.... Yet others may have character pathology that may be the more prominent determinant of drug-taking behavior.... Psychiatric assessment is vitally important for both the population without a prior history of substance abuse and the population of known substance abusers who have a high incidence of psychiatric comorbidity. Treating depression, anxiety, personality disorders, and encephalopathies appropriately may stabilize drug-taking behaviors. (pp. 426–427)

Urine Toxicology Screens

Many experts recommend the use of random urine drug screening as an essential part of the plan of care when drugs with abuse potential are being prescribed, particularly in conjunction with risk stratification efforts that have identified the patients most likely to be vulnerable to problematic drug use, such as those with preexisting substance use disorders or those experiencing an escalation of aberrant drug-taking behavior. Establishing a role for urine drug screening can be challenging for providers, because this screening may be interpreted as demonstrating a lack of trust in the patient's report. Making screens a routine part of clinical care can lessen this discomfort. Open and nonjudgmental communication may also help to ease distrust; for example, a clinician might say, "We'll use this test to help us manage the substance use disorder, which is a potentially lethal disease." Communication that normalizes screening, akin to other disease monitoring strategies, may also be helpful. For example, one might compare urine drug screening for substance use disorders to hemoglobin A1c testing for diabetes monitoring, as an analogy to help reduce the potential shame and embarrassment associated with drug screens.

Prescription Monitoring

Many states have a centralized prescription monitoring program, which can assist the care team in assessing for ongoing aberrant behaviors regarding filling prescriptions from other providers. Routine use of a prescription monitoring program, like urine drug screening, can assist providers in quickly responding to potentially problematic use, thereby protecting patients if loss of control has become an issue. Both urine drug screens and prescription monitoring ought to be discussed transparently with the patient and framed as part of the set of strategies providers will use to help ensure safety.

Harm Reduction

In the palliative care setting, complete remission of a substance use disorder may be unrealistic for many patients. Nonetheless, management of a substance use disorder can be critical to the successful palliation of a patient's symptoms. Although complete abstinence may not be achievable for many reasons (including the possibility that a patient's medical condition may prevent him or her from engaging in a substance use treatment program), it is often possible to reduce some of the negative effects of substance use. Open and honest communication about the patient's substance use disorder, as well as the provision of therapeutic structure and consistency, may help in reducing destructive aberrant behaviors and thereby allow more effective engagement in palliative and disease-directed therapies (Passik and Theobald 2000).

Withdrawal Syndromes

Withdrawal syndromes need to be managed carefully because they can greatly complicate symptom management strategies, can increase the risk of misuse of substances, and can cause significant distress and harm if not effectively addressed. Withdrawal from alcohol and benzodiazepines *can be life threatening,* whereas withdrawal from opioids is highly distressing but generally not dangerous. Withdrawal symptoms should be managed just as aggressively as any other symptoms in palliative care. DSM-5 criteria for opioid and alcohol withdrawal are provided in Table 8–5. Withdrawal can be triggered by dose

Table 8–5. DSM-5 criteria for alcohol withdrawal and opioid withdrawal

DSM-5 criteria for alcohol withdrawal	DSM-5 criteria for opioid withdrawal

A. Cessation of (or reduction in) alcohol use that has been heavy and prolonged.	A. Presence of either of the following:
	  1. Cessation of (or reduction in) opioid use that has been heavy and prolonged (i.e., several weeks or longer).
	  2. Administration of an opioid antagonist after a period of opioid use.

B. Two (or more) of the following, developing within several hours to a few days after the cessation of (or reduction in) alcohol use described in Criterion A:
  1. Autonomic hyperactivity (e.g., sweating or pulse rate greater than 100 bpm).
  2. Increased hand tremor.
  3. Insomnia.
  4. Nausea or vomiting.
  5. Transient visual, tactile, or auditory hallucinations or illusions.
  6. Psychomotor agitation.
  7. Anxiety.
  8. Generalized tonic-clonic seizures.
	B. Three (or more) of the following developing within minutes to several days after Criterion A:
	  1. Dysphoric mood.
	  2. Nausea or vomiting.
	  3. Muscle aches.
	  4. Lacrimation or rhinorrhea.
	  5. Pupillary dilation, piloerection, or sweating.
	  6. Diarrhea.
	  7. Yawning.
	  8. Fever.
	  9. Insomnia.

C. The signs or symptoms in Criterion B cause clinically significant distress or impairment in social, occupational, or other important areas of functioning.	

Table 8–5.   DSM-5 criteria for alcohol withdrawal and opioid withdrawal *(continued)*

DSM-5 criteria for alcohol withdrawal *(cont'd)*

D. The signs or symptoms are not attributable to another medical condition and are not better explained by another mental disorder, including intoxication or withdrawal from another substance.

Specify if:

With perceptual disturbances: This specifier applies in the rare instance when hallucinations (usually visual or tactile) occur with intact reality testing, or auditory, visual, or tactile illusions occur in the absence of a delirium.

Source.   DSM-5 criteria for alcohol withdrawal and opioid withdrawal reprinted from *Diagnostic and Statistical Manual of Mental Disorders*, 5th Edition. Washington, DC, American Psychiatric Association, 2013, pp. 499–500 and 547–548. Used with permission. Copyright © 2013 American Psychiatric Association.

reduction or cessation of use of a substance after a prolonged period of heavy use. In general, patients who have been using a substance consistently for several weeks are at risk of withdrawal, but clinicians should be vigilant for withdrawal even when use is thought to be much less. Patients in the palliative care setting are generally more susceptible to experiencing symptoms of withdrawal, and they may progress quickly from mild to severe symptoms, including delirium. Strategies to manage withdrawal should take into account the patient's goals, current disease state, and prognosis, as well as harm reduction goals with respect to the substance use disorder.

Conclusions and Key Points

- Substance use disorders challenge the management of patients with a comorbid serious medical illness, leading to significant distress for patients, their families, and their providers.

- Risk stratification relies on characterizing aberrant drug-taking behaviors and identifying risk factors for substance use disorders. Several screening instruments can assist with risk stratification for substance use disorders.

- For patients most vulnerable to problematic substance use, urine drug screening and routine use of a controlled substances monitoring database should be part of a comprehensive management plan, to enable early identification and response when concerning behaviors arise.

- The presence or emergence of aberrant behaviors should trigger a careful assessment of their origins, because a variety of conditions, some benign and others dangerous, may give rise to such behaviors.

- An interdisciplinary team is essential for the successful treatment of palliative care patients with substance use disorders.

- Identification and treatment of co-occurring psychiatric illness is an essential element of effective management of substance use disorders in the palliative care setting.

- Withdrawal syndromes need to be recognized and managed carefully in the palliative care patient population.

References

American Psychiatric Association: Diagnostic and Statistical Manual of Mental Disorders, 5th Edition. Arlington, VA, American Psychiatric Association, 2013

American Society of Addiction Medicine: Definitions related to the use of opioids for the treatment of pain: consensus statement of the American Academy of Pain Medicine, the American Pain Society, and the American Society of Addiction Medicine. 2001. Available at: http://www.asam.org/docs/publicy-policy-statements/1opioid-definitions-consensus-2-011.pdf?sfvrsn=0. Accessed July 28, 2015.

American Society of Addiction Medicine: Public policy statement: definition of addiction. 2011. Available at: http://www.asam.org/for-the-public/definition-of-addiction. Accessed July 28, 2015.

Ballantyne JC: Treating pain in patients with drug-dependence problems. BMJ 347:f3213, 2013 24324214

Barclay JS, Owens JE, Blackhall LJ: Screening for substance abuse risk in cancer patients using the Opioid Risk Tool and urine drug screen. Support Care Cancer 22(7):1883–1888, 2014 24563103

Brown RL, Rounds LA: Conjoint screening questionnaires for alcohol and other drug abuse: criterion validity in a primary care practice. Wis Med J 94(3):135–140, 1995 7778330

Childers JW, King LA, Arnold RM: Chronic pain and risk factors for opioid misuse in a palliative care clinic. Am J Hosp Palliat Care 32(6):654–659, 2015 24744398

Chou R, Fanciullo GJ, Fine PG, et al: Opioids for chronic noncancer pain: prediction and identification of aberrant drug-related behaviors: a review of the evidence for an American Pain Society and American Academy of Pain Medicine clinical practice guideline. J Pain 10(2):131–146, 2009 19187890

de Leon J, Susce MT, Murray-Carmichael E: The AmpliChip CYP450 genotyping test: integrating a new clinical tool. Mol Diagn Ther 10(3):135–151, 2006 16771600

Derogatis LR, Morrow GR, Fetting J, et al: The prevalence of psychiatric disorders among cancer patients. JAMA 249(6):751–757, 1983 6823028

Ives TJ, Chelminski PR, Hammett-Stabler CA, et al: Predictors of opioid misuse in patients with chronic pain: a prospective cohort study. BMC Health Serv Res 6:46, 2006 16595013

Kirsh KL, Passik SD: Palliative care of the terminally ill drug addict. Cancer Invest 24(4):425–431, 2006 16777696

Kirsh KL, Ehlenberger E, Huskey A, et al: Exploring rates of abnormal pharmacogenetic findings in a pain practice. J Pain Palliat Care Pharmacother 28(1):28–32, 2014 24601730

Koyyalagunta D, Bruera E, Aigner C, et al: Risk stratification of opioid misuse among patients with cancer pain using the SOAPP-SF. Pain Med 14(5):667–675, 2013 23631401

Ma JD, Horton JM, Hwang M, et al: A single-center, retrospective analysis evaluating the utilization of the Opioid Risk Tool in opioid-treated cancer patients. J Pain Palliat Care Pharmacother 28(1):4–9, 2014 24417217

Michna E, Ross EL, Hynes WL, et al: Predicting aberrant drug behavior in patients treated for chronic pain: importance of abuse history. J Pain Symptom Manage 28(3):250–258, 2004 15336337

Passik SD, Kirsh KL: Managing pain in patients with aberrant drug-taking behaviors. J Support Oncol 3(1):83–86, 2005 15724951

Passik SD, Kirsh KL: Pain in patients with alcohol and drug dependence, in Textbook of Palliative Medicine. Edited by Bruera E, Higginson IJ, Ripamonti C, et al. London, Edward Arnold Publishers, 2006, pp 517–524

Passik SD, Kirsh KL: The interface between pain and drug abuse and the evolution of strategies to optimize pain management while minimizing drug abuse. Exp Clin Psychopharmacol 16(5):400–404, 2008 18837636

Passik SD, Theobald DE: Managing addiction in advanced cancer patients: why bother? J Pain Symptom Manage 19(3):229–234, 2000 10760628

Passik SD, Weinreb HJ: Managing chronic nonmalignant pain: overcoming obstacles to the use of opioids. Adv Ther 17(2):70–83, 2000 11010058

Passik SD, Kirsh KL, Whitcomb L, et al: Pain clinicians' rankings of aberrant drug-taking behaviors. J Pain Palliat Care Pharmacother 16(4):39–49, 2002 14635824

Passik SD, Kirsh KL, Webster L: Pseudoaddiction revisited: a commentary on clinical and historical considerations. Pain Manag 1(3):239–248, 2011 24646390

Smith HS, Kirsh KL, Passik SD: Chronic opioid therapy issues associated with opioid abuse potential. J Opioid Manag 5(5):287–300, 2009 19947070

Substance Abuse and Mental Health Services Administration: Results from the 2012 National Survey on Drug Use and Health: Summary of National Findings (NSDUH Series H-46, HHS Publ No SMA-13-4795). Rockville, MD, Substance Abuse and Mental Health Services Administration, 2013

Substance Abuse and Mental Health Services Administration: Substance use disorders. June 17, 2015. Available at: http://www.samhsa.gov/disorders/substance-use%3E. Accessed July 28, 2015.

Weissman DE, Haddox JD: Opioid pseudoaddiction—an iatrogenic syndrome. Pain 36(3):363–366, 1989 2710565

Wu SM, Compton P, Bolus R, et al: The addiction behaviors checklist: validation of a new clinician-based measure of inappropriate opioid use in chronic pain. J Pain Symptom Manage 32(4):342–351, 2006 17000351

Additional Resources

CAGE-AID screening tool. Available at: http://www.integration.samhsa.gov/images/res/CAGEAID.pdf. Accessed November 6, 2015.

National Institute on Alcohol Abuse and Alcoholism. Web site at: http://niaaa.nih.gov.

National Institute on Drug Abuse. Web site at: http://www.drugabuse.gov.

Opioidrisk.com. Web site at: http://www.opioidrisk.com.

Opioid Risk Tool. Available at: The tool itself: https://www.drugabuse.gov/sites/default/files/files/OpioidRiskTool.pdf. Accessed November 6, 2015.

Screener and Opioid Assessment for Patients with Pain. Available at: http://national-paincentre.mcmaster.ca/documents/soapp_r_sample_watermark.pdf. Accessed November 6, 2015.

Center to Advance Palliative Care, Fast Facts

Arnold RM, Claxton R: Fast Fact #244: Screening for opioid misuse and abuse. Available at: https://www.capc.org/fast-facts/244-screening-opioid-misuse-and-abuse/. Accessed July 28, 2015.

Reisfield GM, Paulian GD, Wilson GR: Fast Fact #127: Substance use disorders in the palliative care patient. Available at: https://www.capc.org/fast-facts/127-substance-use-disorders-palliative-care-patient/. Accessed July 28, 2015.

Weissman DE: Fast Fact #68: Is it pain or addiction? Available at: https://www.capc.org/fast-facts/68-it-pain-or-addiction/. Accessed July 28, 2015.

Weissman DE: Fast Fact #69: Pseudoaddiction. Available at: https://www.capc.org/fast-facts/69-pseudoaddiction/. Accessed July 28, 2015.

PART IV

Interventions

9

Psychotherapy

Chapter Overview

Skillful psychotherapy is an indispensable part of the palliative care psychiatrist's skill set. This chapter provides an overview of psychotherapeutic approaches for seriously ill patients, including a general overview of therapeutic effectiveness, a review of supportive psychotherapy approaches, and a more focused discussion of several interventions that have been developed specifically for palliative care populations.

General Approaches: Skillful Communication and Compassionate Presence as Psychotherapy

Arguably, skillful communication and a compassionate presence are necessary elements of any effective psychotherapy, in the sense that healing results from—or at least is made possible by—certain attributes of the clinician's way of being with the patient, separate from the effect of a medication or other somatic intervention. In fact, one major area of expertise that the palliative care subspecialist brings to the care of seriously ill patients involves skillful communication in highly challenging clinical situations. Chochinov et al. (2013) drew on the expertise of a large number of highly experienced psychosocial oncology clinicians to deconstruct the elements of therapeutic effectiveness; the resulting empirical model suggests that skillful use of 1) therapeutic humility, 2) pacing, and 3) presence provide the foundation for effective psychotherapy in palliative care populations.

Communication strategies in palliative care have been widely studied and are beyond the scope of this chapter (see the "Additional Resources" section at the end of this chapter). Many authors have written eloquently about the importance of maintaining a compassionate presence—and the challenges in doing so—in the face of suffering (Back et al. 2009; Halifax 2011). Similarly, the key roles (and limitations) of empathic responsiveness have been explored (Back and Arnold 2013, 2014). Although skillful communication and compassionate presence should be attributes of all clinicians working in palliative care settings, and in the field of medicine for that matter, the mental health specialist brings a broader and deeper skill set, which can include both general supportive therapy approaches and more specific psychotherapy interventions that have been either adapted to or designed for the palliative care setting (Figure 9–1).

Supportive Psychotherapies

For the mental health specialist, supportive psychotherapeutic approaches are generally the starting point for addressing emotional distress in palliative care settings. Supportive therapies are aimed at understanding and normalizing the patient's psychological distress and mobilizing resources for support. Block (2006) has summarized the supportive approach in the following way:

> The primary therapeutic response to psychological distress at the end of life is to listen, using standard communication techniques (using open-ended questions, following up on affectively intense comments made by the patient, tracking with patient associations and expressed concerns, reflecting on patient emotions, etc.). The [clinician], through offering the patient an opportunity to explore fears, concerns and feelings, to reflect on important relationships, past experiences with loss, and hopes for the future, and to share the unique meanings of illness, can provide the patient with a sense of being understood. Being heard and understood, even in sharing the darkest thoughts and feelings, provides a way for the patient to mourn losses, to coun-

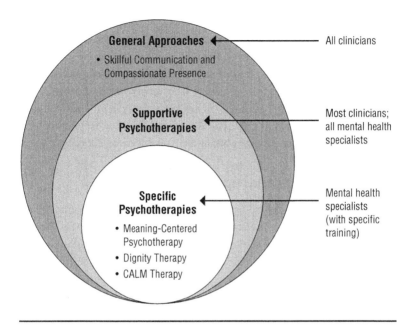

Figure 9–1.   Schema of psychotherapy skill sets in palliative care. CALM = Managing Cancer and Living Meaningfully.

teract the existential isolation of serious illness, to connect with past strengths and coping resources, and to gain a sense of security and mastery.... In general, most terminally ill patients benefit from an approach that combines emotional support, flexibility, appreciation of the patient's strengths, a warm and genuine relationship with the therapist, elements of life-review, and exploration of fears and concerns. The [clinician's] ability to communicate that there are possibilities for meaning, connection, reconciliation, and closure at the end of life may facilitate the patient's ability to accept the approach of death, and to use remaining time well. (pp. 761–762)

Viederman (2008) has described a model that combines supportive and expressive aims, which are sometimes construed as mutually exclusive. Tailored to medically ill patients in crisis, Viederman's approach is potentially useful in the palliative care setting. Interpretative Supportive Dynamic Psychotherapy allows room for the clinician to adopt an interpretive stance, when it is expected to help strengthen a supportive rapport and deepen the patient's experience of being understood. The model relies on active engagement of the therapist (relative to more traditional modes of expressive therapy), with the aim of creating a particular kind of empathic connection, rooted in a shared emotional experience with the patient. Hence, the clinician's approach is aimed at *being with the patient* (as distinct from *acting on the patient*): "being with the patient involves sharing the patient's experience, both present and at times past. Such sharing of experience decreases the sense of isolation and painful loneliness as one struggles with reality" (Viederman 2008, p. 356).

Specific Psychotherapies

Beyond the general use of supportive techniques, a number of specific psychotherapy interventions have been shown to be effective in alleviating psychological distress in palliative care settings. With respect to the treatment of depression, for example, in a 2008 Cochrane review, Akechi et al. (2008) examined the effect of psychotherapy on depressive states in patients with advanced cancer. The review encompassed 10 randomized controlled trials of moderate quality, involving individual- and group-based formats, based on supportive, behavioral, cognitive-behavioral, and problem-solving approaches. In a meta-analysis of a subset of those studies, psychotherapy was associated with significant improvements in depression and general psychological distress, and with marginal improvements in anxiety. These results pertained to depressive states in general; data were not specific to clinically diagnosed depressive disorders (Akechi et al. 2008). A more recent systematic review, more broadly aimed at patients with cancer at all stages of disease, reached a similar conclusion: there is moderate-quality evidence that a variety of psychotherapies can be effective in treating depressive symptoms, but no single intervention can be distinguished on the basis of effectiveness (Li et al. 2012).

Several psychotherapy interventions, described in Table 9–1, have been adapted to or developed specifically for the setting of advanced, life-threatening illness, and palliative care psychiatry providers should be knowledgeable about these. Meaning-Centered Psychotherapy, Dignity Therapy, and Managing Cancer and Living Meaningfully (CALM) are therapy interventions specifically tailored to palliative care settings, and each has shown promise in recent trials, although more research is needed to fully clarify the benefits of these and other psychotherapy interventions for seriously ill patients.

Table 9–1.   Psychotherapies specifically tailored to palliative care settings

Meaning-Centered Psychotherapy (MCPT)	Dignity Therapy (DT)	Managing Cancer and Living Meaningfully (CALM)
	Description	
Brief individual or group therapy	Brief individual therapy	Brief semistructured individual therapy (three to eight sessions)
For patients with terminal illness	For patients with terminal illness	For patients with advanced cancer
Grounded theoretically in existential psychotherapy and the writings and Logotherapy of Viktor Frankl	Derived from an empirical model of dignity	Rooted in relational, attachment, and existential theory
	Aimed at enhancing meaning and purpose	
Typically eight sessions (group) or seven sessions (individual), with mix of didactic, discussion, and experiential methodologies	Typically three sessions, involving semistructured interviews and preparation of a "generativity document"	Addresses four common domains of psychosocial distress:
		• Symptom management; communication with health care providers
Sessions focus conceptually on the generation of meaning, from different sources: creativity, experience, and attitude		• Changes in self; relations with close others
		• Spiritual well-being or sense of meaning and purpose
		• Preparing for future, sustaining hope, facing mortality

Table 9–1.   Psychotherapies specifically tailored to palliative care settings *(continued)*

Meaning-Centered Psychotherapy (MCPT)	Dignity Therapy (DT)	Managing Cancer and Living Meaningfully (CALM)
	Outcomes	
Randomized controlled trial of group format (Breitbart et al. 2010)	*Phase 1 trial* (Chochinov et al. 2005)	*Small qualitative assessment* (Nissim et al. 2012)
Participants randomized to group MCPT vs. Supportive Group Psychotherapy	Patients reported	CALM intervention provides
Posttreatment assessment:	• Small, significant reductions in suffering + depression	• A safe place to process the experience of advanced cancer
• Subjects in MCPT arm reported greater improvements in spiritual well-being and sense of meaning	• Satisfaction with therapy (91%)	• Permission to talk about death and dying
• No significant changes in the control arm	• Heightened sense of dignity (76%)	• Assistance in managing the illness and navigating the health care system
	• Increased sense of purpose (68%)	• Resolution of relational strain
2-month follow-up assessment:	• Heightened sense of meaning (67%)	• Opportunity to "be seen as a whole person" within the health care system
• Improvements in MCPT arm in spiritual well-being and sense of meaning were even more substantial	• Increased will to live (47%)	
• MCPT participants also experienced reductions in anxiety and desire for death	• That it would be of help to their family (81%)	
• No significant changes in the control arm	Family members reported	
	• DT enhanced the patient's dignity (78%)	
	• DT heightened the patient's meaning of life (72%)	
	• The generativity document was a comfort to them (78%)	
	• They would recommend DT to others (95%)	

Table 9–1. Psychotherapies specifically tailored to palliative care settings *(continued)*

Meaning-Centered Psychotherapy (MCPT)	Dignity Therapy (DT)	Managing Cancer and Living Meaningfully (CALM)
	Outcomes *(continued)*	
Randomized Controlled Trial of individual format (Breitbart et al. 2012) Participants randomized to individual MCPT vs. therapeutic massage Posttreatment assessment: • Subjects in MCPT arm reported significantly greater improvements in spiritual well-being, quality of life, symptom burden, and symptom-related distress • No differences in anxiety, depression, or hopelessness 2-month follow-up assessment: • No significant differences between treatment arms	*Randomized controlled trial* (Chochinov et al. 2011) Treatment arms: DT, client-centered care, standard palliative care No significant differences in primary outcomes (global levels of distress in several domains) Secondary outcomes (self-reported end-of-life experiences): • Relative to both control arms: DT significantly more likely to have been helpful (to patient and family); to improve quality of life; to increase sense of dignity; to change family's appreciation for patient • Relative to client-centered care: DT associated with significant improvements in spiritual well-being • Relative to standard palliative care: DT associated with significant improvements in sadness or depression	*Phase 2 trial* (Lo et al. 2014) CALM intervention associated with • Reduced depression • Reduced death anxiety • Improved spiritual well-being • No change in attachment security

Meaning-Centered Psychotherapy

Meaning-Centered Psychotherapy is a short-term intervention with individual and group formats, grounded in the writings and Logotherapy of Viktor Frankl (Breitbart et al. 2004). The treatment seeks to bolster meaning and spiritual well-being in terminally ill patients. In an initial small randomized controlled trial, subjects receiving the group format reported significant improvements in their sense of meaning and spiritual well-being, as well as reductions in anxiety and desire for death, relative to control subjects (Breitbart et al. 2010). A subsequent trial of the individual format showed that participants receiving the meaning-centered intervention experienced significant, but short-lived, improvements in spiritual well-being and quality of life (Breitbart et al. 2012).

Dignity Therapy

Dignity Therapy is a brief individual psychotherapy, derived from an empirical model of dignity, which targets psychosocial and existential distress in terminally ill patients (Chochinov 2002). The intervention incorporates elements of life-review and narrative medicine, through three semistructured interviews and creation of a "generativity document." In a phase 1 trial, patients and families reported high levels of satisfaction with the intervention, as well as broad improvements in sense of dignity, purpose, and meaning (Chochinov et al. 2005). In a follow-up multi-site randomized controlled trial, participants receiving Dignity Therapy reported significant improvements in quality of life, sense of dignity, and spiritual well-being, among other outcomes, relative to matched control subjects. Of note, there were no significant differences in the primary outcome: global levels of distress in several domains (Chochinov et al. 2011). Finally, a recent small, open-label randomized controlled trial of Dignity Therapy was associated with significant reductions in depression at 4 and 15 days posttreatment, and significant reductions in anxiety up to 30 days posttreatment (Julião et al. 2013, 2014).

Managing Cancer and Living Meaningfully

CALM is a brief, semistructured individual psychotherapy that addresses four common domains of psychosocial distress in patients with advanced cancer: 1) symptom management and communication with health care providers; 2) changes in self and relations with close others; 3) spiritual well-being or the sense of meaning and purpose; and 4) preparing for the future, sustaining hope, and facing mortality (Nissim et al. 2012). In a recent phase 2 trial, the CALM intervention was associated with significant reductions in depressive symptoms and death anxiety, and significant increases in spiritual well-being (Lo et al. 2014).

Conclusions and Key Points

- Effective specialist-level palliative care often hinges on skillful communication in highly charged or complex clinical situations.

- Many palliative care providers will have advanced skills in supportive psychotherapy approaches, and the mental health specialist often brings the skill set of an expert, using specific psychotherapy approaches that have been developed for or adapted to the palliative care setting.

- A variety of psychotherapy interventions have been shown to be effective in addressing various dimensions of psychosocial distress in palliative care settings, but data do not support the selection of one modality over another.

- Meaning-Centered Psychotherapy, Dignity Therapy, and CALM therapy have been developed specifically for the setting of advanced, life-threatening illness, and each has shown promise in trials.

- More research is needed to fully clarify the benefits of these and other psychotherapy interventions for seriously ill patients.

References

Akechi T, Okuyama T, Onishi J, et al: Psychotherapy for depression among incurable cancer patients. Cochrane Database Syst Rev (2):CD005537, 2008 18425922

Back AL, Arnold RM: "Isn't there anything more you can do?" When empathic statements work, and when they don't. J Palliat Med 16(11):1429–1432, 2013 24073721

Back AL, Arnold RM: "Yes it's sad, but what should I do?" Moving from empathy to action in discussing goals of care. J Palliat Med 17(2):141–144, 2014 24359216

Back AL, Bauer-Wu SM, Rushton CH, et al: Compassionate silence in the patient-clinician encounter: a contemplative approach. J Palliat Med 12(12):1113–1117, 2009 19698026

Block SD: Psychological issues in end-of-life care. J Palliat Med 9(3):751–772, 2006 16752981

Breitbart W, Gibson C, Poppito SR, et al: Psychotherapeutic interventions at the end of life: a focus on meaning and spirituality. Can J Psychiatry 49(6):366–372, 2004 15283531

Breitbart W, Rosenfeld B, Gibson C, et al: Meaning-centered group psychotherapy for patients with advanced cancer: a pilot randomized controlled trial. Psychooncology 19(1):21–28, 2010 19274623

Breitbart W, Poppito S, Rosenfeld B, et al: Pilot randomized controlled trial of individual meaning-centered psychotherapy for patients with advanced cancer. J Clin Oncol 30(12):1304–1309, 2012 22370330

Chochinov HM: Dignity-conserving care—a new model for palliative care: helping the patient feel valued. JAMA 287(17):2253–2260, 2002 11980525

Chochinov HM, Hack T, Hassard T, et al: Dignity therapy: a novel psychotherapeutic intervention for patients near the end of life. J Clin Oncol 23(24):5520–5525, 2005 16110012

Chochinov HM, Kristjanson LJ, Breitbart W, et al: Effect of dignity therapy on distress and end-of-life experience in terminally ill patients: a randomised controlled trial. Lancet Oncol 12(8):753–762, 2011 21741309

Chochinov HM, McClement SE, Hack TF, et al: Health care provider communication: an empirical model of therapeutic effectiveness. Cancer 119(9):1706–1713, 2013 23341092

Halifax J: The precious necessity of compassion. J Pain Symptom Manage 41(1):146–153, 2011 21123027

Julião M, Barbosa A, Oliveira F, et al: Efficacy of dignity therapy for depression and anxiety in terminally ill patients: early results of a randomized controlled trial. Palliat Support Care 11(6):481–489, 2013 23506744

Julião M, Oliveira F, Nunes B, et al: Efficacy of dignity therapy on depression and anxiety in Portuguese terminally ill patients: a phase II randomized controlled trial. J Palliat Med 17(6):688–695, 2014 24735024

Li M, Fitzgerald P, Rodin G: Evidence-based treatment of depression in patients with cancer. J Clin Oncol 30(11):1187–1196, 2012 22412144

Lo C, Hales S, Jung J, et al: Managing Cancer And Living Meaningfully (CALM): phase 2 trial of a brief individual psychotherapy for patients with advanced cancer. Palliat Med 28(3):234–242, 2014 24170718

Nissim R, Freeman E, Lo C, et al: Managing Cancer and Living Meaningfully (CALM): a qualitative study of a brief individual psychotherapy for individuals with advanced cancer. Palliat Med 26(5):713–721, 2012 22042225

Viederman M: A model for interpretative supportive dynamic psychotherapy. Psychiatry 71(4):349–358, 2008 19152284

Additional Resources

Back A, Arnold R, Tulsky J: Mastering Communication With Seriously Ill Patients: Balancing Honesty With Empathy and Hope. New York, Cambridge University Press, 2009

Chochinov HM: Dignity Therapy: Final Words for Final Days. New York, Oxford University Press, 2011

Cohen ST, Block S: Issues in psychotherapy with terminally ill patients. Palliat Support Care 2:181–189, 2004

Dignity in Care. Web site at: http://www.dignityincare.ca/en.

Halifax J: Being With Dying: Cultivating Compassion and Fearlessness in the Presence of Death. Boston, MA, Shambhala Publications, 2008

Irwin SA, Fairman N, Montross LP: UNIPAC 2: Alleviating Psychological and Spiritual Pain. UNIPAC Self Study Program, 4th Edition. Edited by Storey CP Jr. Glenview, IL, American Academy of Hospice and Palliative Medicine, 2012. Available at: http://www.aahpm.org/resources/default/unipac-4th-edition.html. Accessed July 28, 2015.

Rodin G: Individual psychotherapy for the patient with advanced disease, in Handbook of Psychiatry in Palliative Medicine, 2nd Edition. Edited by Chochinov HM, Breitbart W. New York, Oxford University Press, 2009, pp 443–453

Spiegel D, Leszcz M: Group psychotherapy and the terminally ill, in Handbook of Psychiatry in Palliative Medicine, 2nd Edition. Edited by Chochinov HM, Breitbart W. New York, Oxford University Press, 2009, pp 490–503

VITALtalk. Web site at: http://www.vitaltalk.org.

Pain Management and Psychopharmacology

Chapter Overview

This chapter provides a basic overview of the nomenclature, classification, and general approach to pain management as foundational knowledge for psychiatrists who contribute to pain management in palliative care. The chapter focuses in particular on the use of psychotropic medications as "adjuvant analgesics" in pain management in palliative care settings. In most cases, psychotropic medications are used to complement opioid therapies and other adjuvant pain management approaches, which tend to be the mainstays of treatment. The chapter concludes with clinically focused reviews of evidence supporting the use of psychotropic medication in chronic noncancer pain management and in cancer pain conditions.

Physical Symptom Relief as a Core Tenet of Palliative Care

Expertise in providing relief from physical symptoms is a core tenet of palliative care. The World Health Organization (2015) emphasizes this in its definition of palliative care, the first element of which is the "relief from pain and other distressing symptoms" (see Table 1–1 in Chapter 1, "Palliative Care 101"). Similarly, as discussed in Chapter 1, Cicely Saunders's work emphasized the alleviation of pain as one of the central aims of caring for patients with advanced cancer. In her work one can find the roots of several modern tenets of effective pain management: 1) that a patient's self-report of pain is to be believed, 2) that the treatment plan should be anchored by a comprehensive and iterative assessment, 3) that opioid medications can be used safely at high doses, and 4) that medication should be provided on an around-the-clock basis (Clark 1999).

Although opioid medications provide the cornerstone of pain management for many types of physical pain syndromes, there are many clinical situations in which opioid therapy alone may not be fully effective in achieving adequate pain control, and there are some pain conditions for which opioids should not even be considered as first-line therapy. In such contexts, effective use of nonopioid drug therapies can be critically important, and of these, psychotropic medications often play a substantial role in pain management. Likewise, nonpharmacological approaches, which can take several different forms, have high rates of success in many conditions. Interventional therapies such as nerve blocks, neuroaugmentation, and implantable drug delivery, provided by subspecialists in pain medicine, can provide dramatic and long-lasting benefit in some conditions. Similarly, a number of psychosocial treatments have been deployed as adjuncts to medication therapy in comprehensive approaches to pain management; hypnotherapy (Elkins et al. 2007; Liossi et al. 2006) and cognitive therapy (Eccleston et al. 2002), for example, both have evidence supporting their effectiveness in providing pain relief in some conditions, although the quality of evidence is mixed (Johannsen et al. 2013; Syrjala et al. 2014). Even in cancer populations, psychological interventions such as skills training, education, and supportive-expressive therapy have been associated with significant reductions in cancer pain, in addition to other positive outcomes (Sheinfeld Gorin et al. 2012).

Hence, the approach to pain management in the palliative care setting is often broad and multimodal, drawing on expertise from different disciplines. Although the palliative medicine subspecialist typically takes the lead in directing treatment aimed at pain relief in palliative care settings, there are a number of ways in which psychiatrists can contribute to pain management, as shown in Table 10–1. For example, identifying and addressing coexisting psychiatric conditions (e.g., affective disorders, problems with anxiety) is an im-

Table 10–1.   Roles for psychiatrists in the management of pain in palliative care

Assessing and managing comorbid psychiatric illness (affective disorders, anxiety disorders, psychotic disorders, etc.)

Assessing and managing substance use disorders

Guiding use of psychotropic adjuvant analgesic medication (primarily antidepressants and antiepileptic drugs)

Ensuring optimal use of psychotherapeutic interventions (generally through referral to psychologists and other skilled therapists)

portant complement to traditional drug therapy approaches. Similarly, in chronic pain management there is often a need for help with addressing comorbid substance use disorders.

Pain: The Fundamentals

Definition and Classification

Most contemporary attempts to define *pain* make reference to a combined physical and emotional experience, underscoring the fact that traditional dualities between mind and body tend to lose their explanatory power with respect to the experience of pain. The International Association for the Study of Pain (2012), for example, defines *pain* as "an unpleasant sensory and emotional experience associated with actual or potential tissue damage, or described in terms of such damage." Put more simply, the experience of pain has both physical and psychological components. Among the psychological components, there are elements of emotion and affect, as well as perceptual and interpretive dimensions, which together contribute to the experience of pain.

Pain can be categorized along several variables, and common pain phenomena are defined in Table 10–2. *Acute pain* results from a discrete stimulus that activates specific pain receptors. Typically, acute pain has a physiological or protective role. By contrast, *chronic pain* tends not to be associated with any clearly identifiable event or condition, its duration is often indeterminate (and generally longer than 3 months), and it tends to result from pathological damage to nerves.

Table 10–2.   Nomenclature of common terms in pain management

Pain	An unpleasant sensory and emotional experience associated with actual or potential tissue damage, or described in terms of such damage
Nociceptive pain	Pain that arises from actual or threatened damage to non-neural tissue and is due to the activation of nociceptors
Neuropathic pain	Pain caused by a lesion or disease of the somatosensory nervous system
Allodynia	Pain due to a stimulus that does not normally provoke pain
Analgesia	Absence of pain in response to stimulation that would normally be painful
Hyperalgesia	Increased pain from a stimulus that normally provokes pain
Hypoalgesia	Diminished pain in response to a normally painful stimulus
Paresthesia	An abnormal sensation, whether spontaneous or evoked
Dysesthesia	An unpleasant abnormal sensation, whether spontaneous or evoked

Source.   Adapted from International Association for the Study of Pain 2012.

Another important, and overlapping, distinction can be made on the basis of general physiology. *Nociceptive pain* results from direct stimulation of nerve receptors and "arises from actual or threatened damage to non-neural tissue" (International Association for the Study of Pain 2012). In general, the various forms of acute pain are nociceptive, although chronic pain can also have nociceptive components. Whereas nociceptive pain occurs within a normally functioning somatosensory nervous system, *neuropathic pain* is "caused by a lesion or disease of the somatosensory nervous system" (International Association for the Study of Pain 2012). Most forms of chronic pain involve a high degree of neuropathy. Finally, *mixed pain* has both nociceptive and neuropathic phenomena. Subjectively, patients experience the various kinds of pain in markedly different ways, and treatment approaches differ as well. Table 10–3 describes the differences between nociceptive and neuropathic pain.

Table 10–3.   Distinguishing nociceptive and neuropathic pain

	Nociceptive	Neuropathic
Cause	Direct stimulation of intact nociceptors in somatic or visceral tissues; transmission along normal nerves	Damage to peripheral or central nerve tissue (e.g., compression, transection, infiltration, ischemia, metabolic injury, etc.)
Time pattern	Mostly acute	Often a component of chronic pain
Description	Somatic: sharp, aching, throbbing (easily described) Visceral: gnawing, crampy (often difficult to describe)	Burning, tingling, shooting, stabbing, electrical, numbness
Localization	Somatic: easily localized Visceral: difficult to localize	Generally depends on nerves involved (there are stereotyped patterns—e.g., trigeminal neuralgia)
Tissue injury	Usually apparent	Usually *not* apparent
Drug treatments	Usually responsive to opioids Sometimes helped by adjuvant analgesics	Sometimes responsive to opioids Generally *require* or *rely on* adjuvant analgesics Sometimes require interventional pain techniques

Overview of Pathophysiology

Nociceptive pain results from several linked physiological processes: transduction, conduction, transmission, perception, and modulation (Dharmshaktu et al. 2012). Nociceptors *transduce* painful stimuli (e.g., a burning flame, a pinprick) into signals that are *conducted* along afferent sensory neurons to ascending tracts in the spinal cord. At the terminus of the afferent sensory neuron (i.e., the synapse), the signal is *transmitted* to the ascending tract in the spinal cord. At various levels of the central nervous system (brain stem, thalamus, somatosensory cortex, etc.), *perception* of the pain stimulus occurs. *Modulation* of the pain experience probably occurs throughout the system as well, including via monoamine inputs along the descending tracts. At each level in this process, there are potential targets for intervention, including some for which the psychiatrist may have unique expertise. For example, cognitive therapies can work, in part, through altering the perception of pain; similarly, antidepressant medications (i.e., serotonin-norepinephrine reuptake inhibitors [SNRIs] and tricyclic antidepressants [TCAs]) are believed to influence pain via modulation in descending serotonin or norepinephrine fibers, and possibly also via glutamate and other neurotransmitters in the spinal cord (Ossipov et al. 2014).

The pathophysiology of neuropathic pain is not as well understood. Prolonged physical damage and inflammatory changes in neural tissue appear to result in remodeling of neural architecture and changes in neural chemistry—ultimately producing increased sensitization in peripheral and central circuits, as well as changes that amplify or distort pain perception (Muthuraman et al. 2014).

Approach to Assessment and Management

Effective pain management is rooted in a comprehensive and iterative approach to assessment. Elements of the assessment focus on careful and focused characterization of the location, quality, temporal profile, and severity of pain. Additionally, in palliative care populations, comprehensive pain assessments also encompass broader considerations, such as a review of the underlying disease, attention to nonsomatic dimensions of pain (including psychological and social dimensions), and other elements of pain (Portenoy 2011). Table 10–4 outlines the elements of the assessment of pain in palliative care settings.

Table 10–4.   Elements of the assessment of pain in palliative care settings

Clarification of the underlying disease, planned treatment, expected course, prognosis, and goals of care

Assessment of the chief (pain) complaint
- Characterization of the pain (temporal features, location, intensity, quality, triggers, alleviating factors)
- Formulation of the etiology of pain (causes, types—nociceptive vs. neuropathic, syndromes)

Assessment of the impact of pain
- Effects on physical function and well-being
- Effects on psychological function and well-being
- Effects on role social/interpersonal function and well-being

Assessment of comorbidities
- Medical issues
- Psychiatric issues (depression, anxiety disorders, personality disorders, substance use problems)

Assessment of total pain
- Other physical symptoms
- Emotional, social, spiritual, or existential concerns
- Practical/logistical concerns
- Caregiver issues
- Problems in communication, care coordination, and/or goal setting

Iterative assessment
- Attention to functional outcomes and achievement of goals

Source.   Adapted from Portenoy 2011.

Broadly, the principles of management include reliance on multimodal treatments (pharmacological, interventional, psychotherapeutic, rehabilitative, etc.), the use of a stepwise approach to drug therapy, a focus on functional outcomes, and an emphasis on iterative assessment. With respect to medication strategies, it is useful to divide drug therapies into three broad categories: 1) nonopioid analgesics, such as acetaminophen and nonsteroidal anti-inflammatory drugs; 2) opioid analgesics; and 3) adjuvant analgesic medications, a diverse group of agents from different classes, with primary actions other than analgesia, which may play a complementary role in pain management. Importantly for psychiatrists, antidepressant and antiepileptic drugs (AEDs) are commonly used as adjuvant analgesics.

The World Health Organization's (1996) pain relief ladder is a widely used framework to guide drug therapy for pain management (Figure 10–1). Treatment decisions are driven by the severity of pain: for pain that is mild, nonopioid analgesics are generally the first-line medication strategy. Adjuvant medications can be used as well, often targeting a particular etiology of pain (e.g., steroids for bone pain). On the second step of the ladder, if the initial strategy is ineffective or if pain is moderate at the time of presentation, opioid therapy is the mainstay of treatment. Depending on the temporal pattern of the pain, opioids are generally provided on a scheduled basis (around the clock) as well as on an as-needed basis for breakthrough pain. Nonopioid and adjuvant analgesics are often provided in combination with opioids. On the third step of the ladder, if pain persists or is severe, treatment entails preferential use of a pure opioid drug such as morphine or hydromorphone. Here again, nonopioid analgesics and adjuvant medications are often combined with opioids as part of a broad drug treatment approach. When used appropriately, the stepladder approach is reported to achieve significant relief in 45%–100% of patients with cancer pain (Azevedo São Leão Ferreira et al. 2006).

Use of Psychotropic Medication in Chronic Noncancer Pain Management

Chronic pain is a common and troublesome condition, accounting for a major portion of disability in the United States and worldwide. In 2011, the Institute of Medicine estimated that chronic pain conditions affect well over 100 million Americans, with economic costs in the range of $600 billion annually. For the foreseeable future, the burden of disease from chronic pain is likely to continue to grow, because pain disproportionately affects the elderly, and this segment of the population continues to grow. The management of chronic pain has become a significant area of focus over the past decade: the U.S. Congress, in fact, designated the period from 2001 to 2010 as the "Decade of Pain Control and Research." During roughly the same period, there were marked

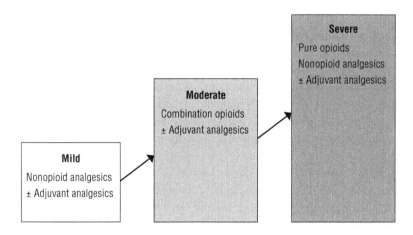

Nonopioid analgesics (e.g., ASA, acetaminophen, NSAIDs)
Combination opioids (e.g., acetaminophen/hydrocodone, acetaminophen/codeine, acetaminophen/oxycodone)
Pure opioids (e.g., morphine, hydromorphone, oxycodone, fentanyl, hydromorphone)
Adjuvant analgesics (e.g., steroids, SNRIs, TCAs, antiepileptic drugs)

Figure 10–1. World Health Organization analgesic ladder for medication management of pain. ASA=acetylsalicylic acid (aspirin); NSAIDs=nonsteroidal anti-inflammatory drugs; SNRIs=serotonin-norepinephrine reuptake inhibitors; TCAs=tricyclic antidepressants.

Source. Adapted from World Health Organization 1996.

increases in opioid sales and abuse, as well as a threefold increase in opioid deaths (Centers for Disease Control and Prevention 2011)—illustrating the major clinical, social, public health, and political ramifications to addressing chronic pain.

The term *chronic pain* is used nonspecifically to refer to a number of different clinical entities. Chronic pain generally occurs in conditions that are not associated with reduced survival, which distinguishes the context of chronic pain management from pain management in more traditional palliative care settings, such as in cancer pain or AIDS. The most common syndromes of chronic pain in the United States include chronic low back pain, diabetic peripheral neuropathy, migraine headaches, arthritis, and fibromyalgia. In most cases, the management of pain in such conditions is grounded (at least initially) in efforts at disease modification.

Highlighting the importance of psychiatric involvement, chronic pain is conceptualized as a "disease of the brain," and approaches to management are increasingly rooted in the biopsychosocial model of disease. Furthermore, chronic pain has a high comorbidity with psychiatric conditions; numerous studies have shown that depression, anxiety disorders, and substance use disorders are overrepresented in various chronic pain conditions, and some research suggests a bidirectional relationship between chronic pain and psychiatric illness (Dharmshaktu et al. 2012; Howe and Sullivan 2014). Finally, there have been long-standing concerns around the safety of opioids in chronic pain management, and a number of investigations have called into question their efficacy in this setting (Ballantyne and Shin 2008; Noble et al. 2010). In fact, for many types of chronic pain, psychotropic medications—not opioids—are considered first-line therapy.

Antidepressants

In general, SNRIs, TCAs, and AEDs appear to have efficacy for many syndromes of chronic pain—independent of their impact on psychiatric disease—and these are often considered first-line drug treatments (Attal et al. 2010; Dworkin et al. 2007; Moulin et al. 2007). Table 10–5 summarizes current evidence supporting the use of antidepressant medications in chronic pain conditions. A 2010 Cochrane review reported efficacy with TCAs and venlafaxine in several different forms of neuropathy (diabetic peripheral neuropathy and postherpetic neuralgia, in particular). Both TCAs and venlafaxine had a strikingly low number needed to treat (NNT), of approximately 3 (Saarto and Wiffen 2007). In contrast to the TCAs and SNRIs, there appears to be little role for selective serotonin reuptake inhibitors (SSRIs) as analgesics for chronic pain; studies indicate that they are either ineffective or inferior to TCAs or SNRIs. Similarly, there are limited data to support the use of antidepressants (of all types) as analgesics in HIV neuropathy, chemotherapy-associated neuropathy, spinal cord injury, and phantom limb pain (Dharmshaktu et al. 2012; Drug and Therapeutics Bulletin 2012; Saarto and Wiffen

2007), although in practice the SNRIs and TCAs are often tried for these specific neuropathies, too.

Antiepileptic Drugs

A number of AEDs are currently used in the management of neuropathic pain, although the evidence supporting their use is mixed, and many of these agents are associated with well-known risks. In a 2013 Cochrane review of the analgesic efficacy of AEDs for neuropathic pain and fibromyalgia, no studies provided first-tier data, and overall there was a lack of quality evidence for most drugs in most types of neuropathic pain and fibromyalgia. However, the gabapentinoids (gabapentin and pregabalin) had second-tier evidence for effectiveness in neuropathic pain and postherpetic neuralgia. NNTs ranged from 4 to 10 for the outcome of 50% reduction in pain from baseline. Pregabalin also had evidence of effectiveness for central neuropathic pain and fibromyalgia (Wiffen et al. 2013). Table 10–5 includes a summary of current evidence regarding the role of AEDs in chronic pain conditions.

Use of Psychotropic Medication in Cancer Pain Management

Surveys indicate that 19%–39% of patients with cancer experience neuropathic pain (Bennett et al. 2012). In cancer, neuropathy may result from direct tumor involvement of neural tissue, or it may be caused by acute or chronic effects of cancer treatment (chemotherapy or radiotherapy). Unsurprisingly, among patients with incurable cancer, the presence of neuropathic pain appears to be associated with reduced performance status and worse physical, cognitive, and social functioning relative to similar patients who experience solely nociceptive pain (Rayment et al. 2013).

Although a number of studies, as noted in the previous section of this chapter, have established the efficacy of antidepressants or AEDs in noncancer neuropathic conditions, there are limited high-quality data examining the use of these agents in cancer-specific neuropathies (Vardy and Agar 2014). As a consequence, clinical practice often relies on extrapolation of data from noncancer settings. A 2011 systematic review reported that AEDs or antidepressants (TCAs or SNRIs), when added to opioid therapy, were likely to produce

Table 10–5.   Psychotropic medications used as adjuvant analgesics

General guidelines

In chronic noncancer pain management:

• Moderate-quality data support the use of SNRIs, TCAs, and gabapentinoids as first-line agents in the treatment of some neuropathies (in particular, diabetic peripheral neuropathy and postherpetic neuralgia) and fibromyalgia.

• Current evidence does not support the use of SSRIs.

• Current evidence does not support the use of antidepressants (of any type) as analgesics in HIV neuropathy, spinal cord injury, or phantom limb pain, although SNRIs and TCAs are often used in practice.

• There is limited evidence supporting the use of other AEDs.

In cancer-related neuropathy:

• Limited high-quality data are available to support the efficacy of antidepressants or AEDs in cancer-specific neuropathies. As a consequence, clinical practice tends to be extrapolated from noncancer settings.

• Gabapentinoids (gabapentin and pregabalin) are reasonable options as first-line adjuvant analgesic agents for cancer-related neuropathy.

• SNRIs and TCAs may have a role in opioid-refractory neuropathic pain, especially when complicated by comorbid depression or anxiety.

Caution is encouraged overall, given the quality of data, potential for adverse effects, and drug-drug interactions in medically vulnerable populations.

Table 10–5.   Psychotropic medications used as adjuvant analgesics *(continued)*

Drug by class	Suggested dosing, titration	Notes
Antidepressants		
SNRIs		Often first-line treatment in diabetic peripheral neuropathy and some other neuropathies (NNT ~ 3–6)
		Favorable side-effect profile relative to TCAs
		Adequate trial requires ~6–8 weeks at therapeutic dose, but some data suggest a rapid neuropathic benefit.
Venlafaxine	75 mg/day PO (extended release)	Neuropathic effect believed to occur at higher end of dose range
	Increase by 75 mg q 1 week (max ~225 mg/day PO)	Many common adverse effects (e.g., insomnia, headache, hypertension)
		Significant discontinuation syndrome; taper to discontinue.
		Extended-release formulation permits once-daily dosing.
Duloxetine	30 mg/day PO	FDA approval for diabetic neuropathy, fibromyalgia, and chronic musculoskeletal pain
	Increase by 30 mg q 1 week (max ~120 mg/day PO)	Doses >60 mg/day do not appear to be more efficacious.
		Many common adverse effects (nausea, somnolence, headache)
		Significant discontinuation syndrome; taper to discontinue.

Table 10–5.   Psychotropic medications used as adjuvant analgesics *(continued)*

Drug by class	Suggested dosing, titration	Notes
Antidepressants (continued)		
TCAs		
Secondary amines (less sedating; less anticholinergic) Desipramine Nortriptyline	10–25 mg PO qhs Increase by 10–25 mg q 3–5 days	Often second-line therapy in neuropathy (after SNRIs), because tolerability is a concern. Good data for efficacy in some forms of neuropathic pain, fibromyalgia, low back pain, and headaches (NNT ~ 3–4). Secondary amines (desipramine, nortriptyline) tend to be better tolerated.
Tertiary amines (more sedating; more anticholinergic) Amitriptyline Imipramine	Usual effective dose ~50–150 mg/day	Concerns include high anticholinergic load (increased risk of delirium); orthostatic hypotension; cardiotoxicity (obtain screening ECG); many drug-drug interactions (TCAs are CYP2D6 substrates; combination with inhibitors will raise dose of TCA). Analgesic doses are often lower than antidepressant doses. Analgesia possible within days, but adequate trial requires 6–8 weeks.
Other antidepressants (SSRIs, bupropion, trazodone, mirtazapine, etc.)		There is insufficient evidence to recommend the use of other antidepressants as adjuvant analgesics.

Table 10–5. Psychotropic medications used as adjuvant analgesics *(continued)*

Drug by class	Suggested dosing, titration	Notes
AEDs		
Gabapentinoids		
Gabapentin	300 mg PO tid Increase by ~300 mg/day q 3 days, to max ~3,600 mg/day (divided tid)	FDA approval for postherpetic neuralgia
Pregabalin	75 mg PO bid After 1 week, increase to 150 mg bid (max ~300 mg bid)	FDA approval for diabetic peripheral neuropathy, fibromyalgia, postherpetic neuralgia, and spinal cord injury neuropathy
Other AEDs (lamotrigine, valproic acid, topiramate, carbamazepine, etc.)		There is insufficient evidence to recommend the use of other AEDs as adjuvant analgesics (see Wiffen et al. 2013).

Note. Dosing guidelines reflect a general initial strategy based on the clinical experience of the authors and current drug references (Micromedex DRUGDEX 2014). Local experts and other resources should be consulted for specific concerns (e.g., dosing strategies in incomplete responders, or dose adjustments in hepatic/renal insufficiency). FDA-labeled indications are included in the table; users should consult with current references for updates. AED=antiepileptic drug; bid=twice daily; CYP=cytochrome P450; ECG=electrocardiogram; FDA=U.S. Food and Drug Administration; max=maximum; NNT=number needed to treat; PO=per oral; q=every; qhs=at bedtime; SNRI=serotonin-norepinephrine reuptake inhibitor; SSRI=selective serotonin reuptake inhibitor; TCA=tricyclic antidepressant; tid=three times daily.

modest reductions in pain within a small number of days; however, the use of adjuvants was also associated with greater exposure to adverse events (Bennett 2011). Similarly, in a more recent systematic review, Jongen et al. (2013) evaluated evidence for efficacy and adverse events associated with drug treatment of neuropathic cancer pain. Overall, the authors concluded, "in patients with neuropathic cancer pain, the beneficial effects of antidepressants, anticonvulsants, opioids, or other adjuvant analgesics greatly outweigh the adverse effects" (p. 587.e1). However, the studies included in the review had major methodological limitations, and overall the quality of evidence was poor: nearly half of the reviewed studies were uncontrolled, and many of the controlled studies did not produce statistically significant differences in efficacy between active and control medications. Nonetheless, the results appear to consistently suggest a benefit from treatment, as well as a relatively low likelihood of harm. Finally, a recent randomized clinical trial of duloxetine demonstrated significant reductions in chemotherapy-induced neuropathic pain relative to placebo (Smith et al. 2013).

Although the data supporting the use of psychotropic medication in cancer pain are limited, some conclusions can be drawn: In general, opioids are first-line medication therapy in cancer pain, whether it is nociceptive, neuropathic, or mixed. Gabapentinoids (gabapentin and pregabalin) can be considered for combination therapy when opioid responsiveness is incomplete. However, if depression or anxiety (or both) are present, SNRIs or TCAs would be preferred. Because of a favorable side-effect profile, SNRIs are often chosen before TCAs. Other AEDs can be considered as third-line adjuvants, if the above strategies are ineffective (Portenoy 2011).

Conclusions and Key Points

- Psychiatrists can have several important roles in pain management in palliative care settings, including managing comorbid psychiatric conditions, assisting with the management of substance use disorders, ensuring that psychotherapeutic interventions are optimized, and directing the use of psychotropic medication as adjuvant analgesics.

- Pain assessment in palliative care settings should be comprehensive and iterative over time, with an emphasis on functional outcomes and quality of life.

- Effective management of pain in palliative care requires multimodal strategies, drawing on expertise from different disciplines.

- Current practice generally favors the use of antiepileptic drugs (especially the gabapentinoids) and/or antidepressant medications (SNRIs or TCAs) in an adjuvant role in the management of neuropathic pain in palliative care populations. However, high-quality data are lacking.

- Caution should be exercised when using antidepressants and/or antiepileptic drugs as adjuvant analgesics, because these agents are associated with a number of common adverse events, particularly among patients with serious illness.

References

Attal N, Cruccu G, Baron R, et al; European Federation of Neurological Societies: EFNS guidelines on the pharmacological treatment of neuropathic pain: 2010 revision. Eur J Neurol 17(9):1113–e88, 2010 20402746

Azevedo São Leão Ferreira K, Kimura M, Jacobsen Teixeira M: The WHO analgesic ladder for cancer pain control, twenty years of use. How much pain relief does one get from using it? Support Care Cancer 14(11):1086–1093, 2006 16761128

Ballantyne JC, Shin NS: Efficacy of opioids for chronic pain: a review of the evidence. Clin J Pain 24(6):469–478, 2008 18574357

Bennett MI: Effectiveness of antiepileptic or antidepressant drugs when added to opioids for cancer pain: systematic review. Palliat Med 25(5):553–559, 2011 20671006

Bennett MI, Rayment C, Hjermstad M, et al: Prevalence and aetiology of neuropathic pain in cancer patients: a systematic review. Pain 153(2):359–365, 2012 22115921

Centers for Disease Control and Prevention: Vital signs: overdoses of prescription opioid pain relievers—United States, 1999–2008. MMWR Morb Mortal Wkly Rep 60(43):1487–1492, 2011 22048730

Clark D: "Total pain," disciplinary power and the body in the work of Cicely Saunders, 1958–1967. Soc Sci Med 49(6):727–736, 1999 10459885

Dharmshaktu P, Tayal V, Kalra BS: Efficacy of antidepressants as analgesics: a review. J Clin Pharmacol 52(1):6–17, 2012 21415285

Drug and Therapeutics Bulletin: An update on the drug treatment of neuropathic pain. Part 1: antidepressants. Drug Ther Bull 50(10):114–117, 2012

Dworkin RH, O'Connor AB, Backonja M, et al: Pharmacologic management of neuropathic pain: evidence-based recommendations. Pain 132(3):237–251, 2007 17920770

Eccleston C, Morley S, Williams A, et al: Systematic review of randomised controlled trials of psychological therapy for chronic pain in children and adolescents, with a subset meta-analysis of pain relief. Pain 99(1–2):157–165, 2002 12237193

Elkins G, Jensen MP, Patterson DR: Hypnotherapy for the management of chronic pain. Int J Clin Exp Hypn 55(3):275–287, 2007 17558718

Howe CQ, Sullivan MD: The missing 'P' in pain management: how the current opioid epidemic highlights the need for psychiatric services in chronic pain care. Gen Hosp Psychiatry 36(1):99–104, 2014 24211157

Institute of Medicine: Relieving Pain in America: A Blueprint for Transforming Prevention, Care, Education, and Research. Washington, DC, National Academy of Sciences, 2011

International Association for the Study of Pain: IASP taxonomy. May 22, 2012. Available at: http://www.iasp-pain.org/Taxonomy. Accessed July 29, 2015.

Johannsen M, Farver I, Beck N, et al: The efficacy of psychosocial intervention for pain in breast cancer patients and survivors: a systematic review and meta-analysis. Breast Cancer Res Treat 138(3):675–690, 2013 23553565

Jongen JL, Huijsman ML, Jessurun J, et al: The evidence for pharmacologic treatment of neuropathic cancer pain: beneficial and adverse effects. J Pain Symptom Manage 46(4):581.e1–590.e1, 2013

Liossi C, White P, Hatira P: Randomized clinical trial of local anesthetic versus a combination of local anesthetic with self-hypnosis in the management of pediatric procedure-related pain. Health Psychol 25(3):307–315, 2006 16719602

Micromedex DRUGDEX (Internet database). Ann Arbor, MI, Truven Health Analytics, 2014. Available at: www.micromedexsolutions.com. Subscription required to view.

Moulin DE, Clark AJ, Gilron I, et al; Canadian Pain Society: Pharmacological management of chronic neuropathic pain—consensus statement and guidelines from the Canadian Pain Society. Pain Res Manag 12(1):13–21, 2007 17372630

Muthuraman A, Singh N, Jaggi AS, et al: Drug therapy of neuropathic pain: current developments and future perspectives. Curr Drug Targets 15(2):210–253, 2014 24093749

Noble M, Treadwell JR, Tregear SJ, et al: Long-term opioid management for chronic noncancer pain. Cochrane Database Syst Rev (1):CD006605, 2010 20091598

Ossipov MH, Morimura K, Porreca F: Descending pain modulation and chronification of pain. Curr Opin Support Palliat Care 8(2):143–151, 2014 24752199

Portenoy RK: Treatment of cancer pain. Lancet 377(9784):2236–2247, 2011 21704873

Rayment C, Hjermstad MJ, Aass N, et al; European Palliative Care Research Collaborative (EPCRC): Neuropathic cancer pain: prevalence, severity, analgesics and impact from the European Palliative Care Research Collaborative-Computerised Symptom Assessment study. Palliat Med 27(8):714–721, 2013 23175513

Saarto T, Wiffen PJ: Antidepressants for neuropathic pain. Cochrane Database Syst Rev (4):CD005454, 2007 17943857

Sheinfeld Gorin S, Krebs P, Badr H, et al: Meta-analysis of psychosocial interventions to reduce pain in patients with cancer. J Clin Oncol 30(5):539–547, 2012 22253460

Smith EM, Pang H, Cirrincione C, et al; Alliance for Clinical Trials in Oncology: Effect of duloxetine on pain, function, and quality of life among patients with chemotherapy-induced painful peripheral neuropathy: a randomized clinical trial. JAMA 309(13):1359–1367, 2013 23549581

Syrjala KL, Jensen MP, Mendoza ME, et al: Psychological and behavioral approaches to cancer pain management. J Clin Oncol 32(16):1703–1711, 2014 24799497

Vardy J, Agar M: Nonopioid drugs in the treatment of cancer pain. J Clin Oncol 32(16): 1677–1690, 2014 24799483

Wiffen PJ, Derry S, Moore RA, et al: Antiepileptic drugs for neuropathic pain and fibromyalgia—an overview of Cochrane reviews. Cochrane Database Syst Rev (11): CD010567, 2013 24217986

World Health Organization: WHO Cancer Pain Relief, With a Guide to Opioid Availability, 2nd Edition. Geneva, World Health Organization, 1996

World Health Organization: WHO definition of palliative care. 2015. Available at: http://www.who.int/cancer/palliative/definition/en/. Accessed July 29, 2015.

Additional Resources

Breitbart W, Passik SD, Casper DJ, et al: Psychiatric aspects of pain management in patients with advanced cancer and AIDS, in Handbook of Psychiatry in Palliative Medicine, 2nd Edition. Edited by Chochinov HM, Breitbart W. New York, Oxford University Press, 2009, pp 384–416

Education in Palliative and End-of-Life-Care for Oncology (EPEC-Oncology). Module 2: Cancer Pain Management. Available at: http://www.cancer.gov/cancertopics/cancerlibrary/epeco. Accessed July 29, 2015.

Kerns RD, Sellinger J, Goodin BR: Psychological treatment of chronic pain. Annu Rev Clin Psychol 7:411–434, 2011

Portenoy RK, El Osta B, Bruera E: Physical symptom management in the terminally ill, in Handbook of Psychiatry in Palliative Medicine, 2nd Edition. Edited by Chochinov HM, Breitbart W. New York, Oxford University Press, 2009, pp 355–383

Weinstein S, Portenoy RK, Harrington SE: UNIPAC 3: Assessing and Treating Pain. UNIPAC Self Study Program, 4th Edition. Edited by Storey CP Jr. Glenview, IL, American Academy of Hospice and Palliative Medicine, 2012. Available at: http://www.aahpm.org/resources/default/unipac-4th-edition.html. Accessed July 29, 2015.

Center to Advance Palliative Care, Fast Facts

Bidar-Sielaff S, Gordon D: Fast Fact #78: Cultural aspects of pain management. Available at: https://www.capc.org/fast-facts/78-cultural-aspects-pain-management/. Accessed July 29, 2015.

Fernandez C, Mehta Z, Espenlaub A, et al: Fast Fact #197: Chemotherapy-induced peripheral neuropathy. Available at: https://www.capc.org/fast-facts/197-chemo-therapy-induced-peripheral-neuropathy/. Accessed July 29, 2015.

Hawley P: Fast Fact #187: Non-tricyclic antidepressants for neuropathic pain. https://www.capc.org/fast-facts/187-non-tricyclic-antidepressants-neuropathic-pain/. Accessed July 29, 2015.

Hepner S, Claxton R: Fast Fact #271: Anti-epileptic drugs for pain. Available at: https://www.capc.org/fast-facts/271-anti-epileptic-drugs-pain/. Accessed July 29, 2015.

King, L, Kishore A, Weissman DE: Fast Fact #49: Gabapentin for neuropathic pain. Available at: https://www.capc.org/fast-facts/49-gapapentin-neuropathic-pain/. Accessed July 29, 2015.

PART V

Pediatric Patients

Children and Adolescents

Chapter Overview

Although much of the content in this book pertains broadly to both adult and pediatric populations, the care of children and adolescents with serious illnesses often raises unique considerations. A child's developmental stage, the importance of family systems, and issues around grieving, for example, warrant special attention in pediatric palliative care. Material in this chapter complements content elsewhere in the book, while adding a focus on issues that are particular to the psychiatric care of children and adolescents in palliative care settings.

Each year in the United States, over 43,000 children die from and approximately 500,000 receive treatment for a life-limiting illness (Hamilton et al. 2013). For these children and their families—just as for adult populations—there is a considerable need for palliative care expertise. In fact, as the field of palliative care has matured over the last two decades, significant progress has been made in expanding the interface between palliative medicine and the care of seriously ill children and adolescents, including increased attention to the need for specialized psychiatric care as an element of comprehensive pediatric palliative care. Treatment by the pediatric palliative care team should be available wherever the patient is receiving care, including in specialty ambulatory care settings, the acute care hospital, the intensive care unit (ICU), and home-based palliative care and hospice settings. Any pediatric patient with a serious illness that is significantly impacting quality of life may benefit from the involvement of a specialist palliative care team; kids with cancer, cystic fibrosis, or muscular dystrophy are common examples. Table 11–1 lists the ideal members of a pediatric palliative care team, which should include a psychiatrist.

Psychiatrist's Role in Pediatric Palliative Care Team

Just as in adult palliative care, the mental health specialist working with pediatric populations brings a unique skill set to the prevention and relief of suffering in seriously ill children and their families. As Wolfe et al. (2011) noted, "The contribution of child psychology and psychiatry, as well as other mental health disciplines, provides specialized knowledge and skills. The specific and unique interventions include: evaluation of the child's psychological status, diagnosis of psychological/psychiatric symptoms and disturbance, psychotherapy and psychotropic medication, and consultation to families and the team" (p. 28).

The psychiatrist's principal role in the pediatric palliative care team is to provide comprehensive assessment and medication treatments for psychiatric symptoms. In addition, in many respects the psychiatrist operates as a coordinator of care, because pediatric mental health interventions are often multimodal and nonpharmacological interventions are numerous. For example, having made a careful diagnostic assessment of anxiety symptoms, the psychiatrist may identify a need for relaxation skills training and recruit a hypnotherapist to lead this element of the treatment plan. The coordination and integration of a variety of assessments and treatment modalities is key to the provision of high-quality, comprehensive child and adolescent palliative care psychiatry. In addition, the psychiatrist is often called on to lend support to other members of the clinical team. The challenge of managing psychiatric symptoms and/or of negotiating complicated family dynamics can frequently

Table 11–1.   Team composition for comprehensive child and adolescent palliative care

Pediatric palliative medicine specialist

Pediatric palliative care nurse practitioner (or advanced practice nurse)

Pediatric palliative care social worker

Child and adolescent palliative care psychiatrist

Psychotherapist (e.g., psychologist, marriage and family therapist, clinical social worker)

Chaplain

Clinical pharmacist

Child-life specialist

Complementary/alternative treatment providers (e.g., hypnotherapist, massage therapist, music therapist, acupuncturist)

become overwhelming for primary care providers, impacting their ability to deliver optimal care. The psychiatrist can alleviate some of the distress shared among members of the clinical team by leading the management of the patient's psychiatric symptoms as well as by providing support to colleagues.

Unique Issues in Pediatric Palliative Care Psychiatry

Communication About Illness

The importance of effective communication in highly challenging clinical situations—arguably one of the hallmark skills in specialist-level palliative care—takes on even greater significance in the care of seriously ill children and adolescents (Fosson and deQuan 1984; Lambert et al. 2008). Children (and their parents) often experience high levels of uncertainty about their illness and the treatments they face, and effective communication helps to form a trustful relationship between providers, patients, and parents, which in turn helps to reduce distress (Beale et al. 2005).

Children should be included in discussions about their health, disease, treatments, and prognosis, and they should be allowed to participate in decision making to the extent that they are able. Communication strategies need to take into account the patient's level of developmental maturity, especially with respect to serious topics such as the expected progression of disease, life expectancy, and risks of treatment (Levetown and American Academy of Pediatrics Committee on Bioethics 2008). Disclosure of information to children—including about the possibility of death—has been found to reduce distress in both patients and parents (Kreicbergs et al. 2004). In discussions of serious medical issues, one should rely on the gentle use of concrete and specific terms and phrases, and avoid euphemisms. For example, "Eventually, you will *die from this disease*" is preferred to "Eventually, you will *pass away.*" Quill et al. (2014, p. 209) suggest the following useful questions to help initiate such discussions:

- "What do you know about what's going on? What would you like to know?"
- "Why do you think this is happening? Do you have some ideas about why you've gotten sick?"
- "Would you like to know what I think is happening to you?"

In such discussions, it is important to carefully clarify the child's responses, to ensure that the conversation does not go beyond his or her expectations or comfort level.

Concept of Death

It is often assumed that children lack the ability to understand or conceptualize death in any sophisticated way, owing to limited life experience and underdeveloped levels of abstract thinking. However, the illness experiences of children with serious diseases—marked by early familiarity with physical suffering, "medicalization" from prolonged hospitalization or other clinical experience, losses in psychosocial and educational spheres, and (often) familiarity with death as both a concept and an actual experience through relationships with other sick children—often contribute to their having a more maturely developed conceptualization of death than their same-age peers (Beale et al. 2005; Schonfeld 1993). Table 11–2 provides general guidance about the concept of death at different developmental stages, as it pertains to strategies for support and communication with children and adolescents.

Table 11–2. Concept of death in children and strategies for palliative care support and communication

Age group	Concept of death/developmental stage	Strategies
Infants (~0–2 years)	No understanding of meaning of death May have awareness that something is wrong	Support maximal contact with loved ones (who provide safety and comfort) Ensure consistency of routines Use concrete language
Toddlers (~2–6 years)	Death is temporary, similar to sleep; may be viewed as a punishment Magical thinking may lead to belief that thoughts or wishes can cause or prevent death, leading to guilt May not have understanding that death can happen to them	Minimize separation from loved ones (who provide safety and comfort) Assess for degree of magical thinking and resulting guilt; correct if needed Ensure consistency of routines Use concrete, specific language (*dying, death, dead, die*); avoid euphemisms (*passing away*)
Children (~6–12 years)	Maturing understanding of death; may develop awareness that they can die Often curious for details about illness and death	Encourage participation in care planning Encourage time with family and peers Use simple cause-effect statements Explore fears Use direct, honest communication to discuss disease, treatments, and prognosis

Table 11–2. Concept of death in children and strategies for palliative care support and communication (*continued*)

Age group	Concept of death/developmental stage	Strategies
Teens (~12–18 years)	Begin to develop a sense of the universal, personal, and specific nature of death Body image and social standing take on increasing importance, and they are seen in connection with illness May begin to develop conception of spiritual or nonphysical aspects of death May develop a desire for a sense of meaning related to illness and death	Encourage time with peers Respect needs for physical and emotional privacy Encourage participation in goal setting and care planning Continue direct, honest communication about disease, treatments, and prognosis

Source.   Adapted from Himelstein et al. 2004.

Attention to Physical and Psychological Symptoms

The relationship between physical and psychological symptoms is often bidirectional: physical problems can produce emotional distress, and psychological problems can produce somatic symptoms. In adults—and perhaps even more so in children and adolescents—the overwhelming emotional experience of being sick can worsen the physical experience of illness. Hence, consistent with Cicely Saunders's conceptualization of total pain, optimal treatment of physical symptoms requires simultaneous attention to the psychiatric dimensions of suffering, and vice versa (Hirsh and Friebert 2014).

Depression

Broadly, the management of depression in children and adolescents is similar to the approach taken with adults. Several important differences warrant mention, however. In terms of the assessment, for example, for the clinician to gather comprehensive data to inform an accurate assessment, a child's subjective report often needs to be complemented by collateral information from parents and other caregivers. Likewise, obtaining details about a family history of mood disorders can greatly aid in assessment. As in seriously ill adults, physical symptoms in children can often masquerade as depression, and the differential diagnosis can be challenging. Table 11–3 provides guidance about the workup for symptoms of depression in medically ill pediatric patients. In children and adolescents, in particular, the following signs and symptoms strongly point to depression: irritability, somatic symptoms (e.g., abdominal pain and gastrointestinal issues, headaches, fatigue), feelings of guilt, poor treatment adherence, apathy, and developmental regression.

Table 11–4 provides an overview of the approach to treating depression in children and adolescents, which parallels the strategies used in adults (see Chapter 3, "Depression"). Clarification of the medical context and goals of care should guide the overall approach to managing depression. The elements of depression management in children, as in adults, should include 1) clarifying and addressing total pain; 2) providing education and general support to the patient and family members; 3) optimizing nonpharmacological strategies, including a variety of psychotherapy approaches; and 4) providing drug treatments in time-limited trials. Nonpharmacological interventions should make

Table 11–3.   Assessment of depression in medically ill pediatric patients

Lab workup

Complete blood count

Complete metabolic panel (including electrolytes, glucose, renal function, liver function, vitamin B_{12}, folate)

Thyroid function tests

Urinalysis

Medication levels, if appropriate

Screening for drugs of abuse

If warranted, head and spine imaging and electroencephalogram

Medication review

Corticosteroids

Opioids

Benzodiazepines

Interferon

Interleukin-2

Chemotherapies

Other contributing factors

Uncontrolled physical symptoms (especially pain, shortness of breath, nausea/vomiting)

Central nervous system (CNS) disease (primary CNS solid tumors, metastases to the brain, CNS lymphoma)

Loss of role identity (e.g., as sibling, student, athlete)

Social isolation and peer abandonment

Physical disfigurement (e.g., hair loss, weight loss/gain)

Source.   Adapted from Pao and Weiner 2011.

Table 11–4. Overview of the treatment of depression in children and adolescents

Address total pain

In particular, manage physical symptoms aggressively.

Leverage expertise of interdisciplinary team.

Optimize psychotherapy and nonpharmacological interventions

A variety of psychotherapy approaches have efficacy in depression in children, and these are sometimes preferable to patients and families.

Provide medication treatment

Should be guided by prognosis and goals of care:

Prognosis ≤6 months:
• Consider psychostimulants as first-line therapy.

Prognosis >6 months:
• Consider typical antidepressants as first-line therapy.
• Titrate aggressively to expected therapeutic dose.
• May see improvement within weeks, but adequate trial requires ~ 8 weeks.

use of specially trained clinicians on the palliative care team, such as child-life specialists, clinical social workers, and psychologists (Powers 1999; Spirito and Kazak 2006). Nonpharmacological interventions may also include play therapy and expressive arts–based therapies, which can be effective at many developmental stages, starting with the young child (Kreitler et al. 2004). Talk-based therapies are often a good fit for more articulate and mature children (March et al. 2007). Bright light therapy, which has been shown to alleviate symptoms of depression in adults, can also play a role in managing depression in pediatric populations (Lieverse et al. 2011; Swedo et al. 1997). Drug treatments for depression in children, described in Table 11–5, are essentially the same as those in adults, although dose adjustments are often necessary.

Anxiety

Both symptoms and disorders of anxiety are highly prevalent in medically ill children and adolescents, with reported rates between 15% and 60% across a

Table 11–5. Drug treatments for depression in children and adolescents

Drug by class	Suggested dosing, titration	Notes
SSRIs		All antidepressants carry a black box warning regarding possible increase of suicidal ideation Often have sexual side effects Adequate trial requires ~6–8 weeks at therapeutic dose
Citalopram	5–20 mg/day PO Increase by 5–20 mg/day q 1–2 weeks; max: ~40 mg/day PO	Generally well tolerated Common adverse effects: dry mouth, GI symptoms, insomnia Few drug-drug interactions Taper to discontinue, when possible Risk of QTc prolongation at doses >40 mg/day Available routes: PO (tabs, liq)
Escitalopram	2.5–10 mg/day PO Increase by 5–10 mg/day q 1–2 weeks; max: ~20 mg/day PO	Generally well tolerated Common adverse effects: dry mouth, GI symptoms, insomnia Few drug-drug interactions Taper to discontinue, when possible Available routes: PO (tabs, liq)
Sertraline	12.5–50 mg/day PO Increase by 50 mg/day q 1–2 weeks; max: ~200 mg/day PO	Generally well tolerated Common adverse effects: dry mouth, GI symptoms, insomnia Few drug-drug interactions Taper to discontinue, when possible Available routes: PO (tabs, liq)

Table 11–5.   Drug treatments for depression in children and adolescents *(continued)*

Drug by class	Suggested dosing, titration	Notes
SSRIs *(continued)*		
Fluoxetine	5–10 mg/day PO Increase by 10–20 mg/day q 1–2 weeks; max: ~40 mg/day PO	Many drug-drug interactions Wide dose range: 5–80 mg/day Do not need to taper to discontinue (very long half-life) May be activating in some patients Available routes: PO (tabs, caps, liq)
Paroxetine	5–10 mg/day PO Increase by 10–20 mg/day q 1–2 weeks; max: ~40 mg/day PO	Common adverse effects: dry mouth, GI symptoms, sedation Many drug-drug interactions Most anticholinergic of the antidepressants Significant discontinuation syndrome (very short half-life); taper to discontinue; use caution when oral route is unreliable Available routes: PO (tabs, liq)
SNRIs		All antidepressants carry a black box warning regarding possible increase of suicidal ideation. Often have sexual side effects Adequate trial requires ~6–8 weeks at therapeutic dose

Table 11–5.   Drug treatments for depression in children and adolescents (*continued*)

Drug by class	Suggested dosing, titration	Notes
SNRIs (*continued*)		
Venlafaxine	12.5–75 mg/day PO (extended release) Increase by 75 mg/day q 1 week; max: ~225 mg/day PO	Many common adverse effects (e.g., insomnia, headache, hypertension) Effective in neuropathic pain (higher doses) Significant discontinuation syndrome (very short half-life); taper to discontinue; use caution when oral route is unreliable Extended-release formulation permits daily dosing Available routes: PO (tabs, caps)
Desvenlafaxine	25–50 mg/day PO May increase after 1 week to 50 mg/day	Many common adverse effects (e.g., nausea, insomnia, anxiety) Major active metabolite of venlafaxine; presumably shares efficacy with depression, anxiety, and neuropathic pain Available routes: PO (tabs)
Duloxetine	20–30 mg/day PO Increase by 30 mg/day q 1 week; max: ~120 mg/day PO	Many common adverse effects Effective in neuropathic pain Doses >120 mg/day rarely more effective Significant discontinuation syndrome; taper to discontinue; use caution when oral route is unreliable Available routes: PO (caps)

Table 11–5. Drug treatments for depression in children and adolescents *(continued)*

Drug by class	Suggested dosing, titration	Notes
Miscellaneous antidepressants		
Bupropion	XL formulation: 75–150 mg PO qam Increase to 300 mg PO qam after ~1 week; max: ~450 mg PO qam	Weak norepinephrine and dopamine reuptake inhibitor Contraindicated with seizures or eating disorders Mild stimulant effect: useful in patients with low energy, but may cause insomnia May improve concentration May augment antidepressant effect and reduce sexual side effect of SSRIs Multiple formulations available (IR, SR, XL); XL formulation permits once-daily dosing Available routes: PO (tabs, caps)
Mirtazapine	7.5–15 mg PO qhs Increase by 15 mg q 1–2 weeks; max: ~45 mg PO qhs	Exact mechanism of action unknown (increases central serotonergic and noradrenergic activity) At lower end of dose range, causes sedation and stimulates appetite; useful in patients with insomnia and anorexia Causes orthostatic hypotension Available routes: PO (tabs, ODT)

Table 11–5. Drug treatments for depression in children and adolescents *(continued)*

Drug by class	Suggested dosing, titration	Notes
Psychostimulants		
Methylphenidate	2.5 mg PO bid (at 8 A.M. and 2 P.M.) Titrate daily by 2.5 mg bid, to maximum tolerated effective dose Max: ~ 30 mg PO bid	Rapid antidepressant effect Consider first line when prognosis ≤6 months May cause or worsen anxiety, motor tics, visual hallucinations May cause or worsen insomnia May stimulate appetite Usual effective dose ≤20 mg bid (doses >30 mg/day usually not necessary) Available routes: PO (tabs, caps, liq)
Dextroamphetamine/ amphetamine	2.5 mg PO bid (at 8 A.M. and 2 P.M.) Titrate daily by 2.5 mg bid, to maximum tolerated effective dose Max: ~20 mg PO bid	May cause or worsen anxiety, motor tics, visual hallucinations May cause or worsen insomnia May stimulate appetite Usual effective dose ≤20 mg bid (doses >30 mg/day usually not necessary) Available routes: PO (tabs, caps, liq)

Note.   Dosing guidelines reflect a general initial strategy based on the clinical experience of the authors and current drug references (Micromedex DRUGDEX 2014; Stahl 2014). Local experts and other resources should be consulted for specific concerns (e.g., dosing strategies in incomplete responders, or dose adjustments in hepatic/renal insufficiency). All first-line antidepressants in this table (SSRIs, SNRIs, bupropion, mirtazapine) have an U.S. Food and Drug Administration indication for major depressive disorder. For other drugs on this table, treatment of major depression is off-label.   bid=twice daily; caps=capsules; GI=gastrointestinal; IR=immediate release; liq=liquid; max=maximum; ODT=orally disintegrating tablet; PO=per oral; q=every; qam =every morning; qhs=bedtime; SNRI=serotonin-norepinephrine reuptake inhibitor; SR=sustained release; SSRI=selective serotonin reuptake inhibitor; tabs=tablets; XL=extended release.

range of illnesses (Chavira et al. 2008). As in the adult population, physical symptoms and anxiety are often closely intertwined: anxiety can be precipitated by physical symptoms (or by the anticipation of physical symptoms), and anxiety can amplify the experience of physical symptoms, making them more difficult to treat. Anxiety can also transform routine parts of patient care, such as venipuncture or removal of dressings, into highly distressful experiences. Physical conditions that commonly contribute to anxiety symptoms include metabolic derangements, pulmonary disease, neurological disease (including delirium, seizures, and sequelae of traumatic brain injury), endocrinology disorders, cardiac disease, and cancer. Although the workup and differential diagnosis of anxiety in children closely parallels the approach outlined for adults in Chapter 4, "Anxiety," the diagnosis of anxiety in a child or adolescent can be quite challenging, and it is frequently useful to seek consultation with a child and adolescent psychiatrist in such cases.

The approach to treating anxiety uses the same strategies emphasized in the previous section with respect to depression (regarding addressing total pain, clarifying the context and goals of care, optimizing nonpharmacological interventions, and using time-limited trials for drug treatment). Table 11–6 gives an overview of the approach to managing anxiety symptoms, and Table 11–7 provides details about medication therapies.

Insomnia

Insomnia is very common in medically ill children, especially in those with life-threatening illnesses. For example, sleep disturbances have been reported in up to 40% of patients with cystic fibrosis (Naqvi et al. 2008) and in 30%–60% of children with cancer (Collins et al. 2002). Pain is a common contributor to insomnia: in the pediatric pain clinic setting, up to 70% of patients report sleep issues (Lewin and Dahl 1999). Common causes of pediatric insomnia are detailed in Table 11–8.

The assessment of insomnia in children is similar to assessment in adults (see Chapter 7, "Insomnia"). However, in assessments of children, it is particularly important to make use of parents and caregivers as informants, and also to understand sleep requirements in the context of the child's particular developmental stage. Before initiating treatment for insomnia in a child, it is important to ensure that the goals for sleep improvement align with what would be

Table 11–6.   Overview of the treatment of anxiety in children and
adolescents

Address total pain

In particular, manage physical symptoms aggressively.

Optimize reliance on interdisciplinary team.

Optimize psychotherapy and nonpharmacological interventions

A variety of psychotherapy approaches have efficacy in anxiety in children, and
these are sometimes preferable to patients and families.

Provide medication treatment

Should be guided by prognosis and goals of care:

Prognosis ≤6 months:
- In mild to moderate anxiety, consider prn trazodone or gabapentin.
- In severe anxiety, consider prn lorazepam and/or scheduled clonazepam.

Prognosis >6 months:
- In mild to moderate anxiety, use scheduled SSRI/SNRI and consider prn
  trazodone or gabapentin.
- In severe anxiety, use scheduled SSRI/SNRI and consider prn lorazepam.
- Titrate antidepressant aggressively to expected therapeutic dose.
- Adequate trial requires ~8 weeks.

Note.   prn=as needed; SNRI=serotonin-norepinephrine reuptake inhibitor; SSRI=selective
serotonin reuptake inhibitor.

expected developmentally and with the patient's baseline sleep experience.
Sleep diaries completed by parents or patients can aid the assessment. The
BEARS tool is a screening instrument that can help guide assessment of sleep
problems in the pediatric palliative care population (Owens and Dalzell 2005).
(BEARS is an acronym for **B**edtime Issues, **E**xcessive Daytime Sleepiness,
Night **A**wakenings, **R**egularity and Duration of Sleep, and **S**noring.)

Nonpharmacological approaches, detailed in Table 11–9, are often suffi-
cient to manage insomnia in children, and treatment should always begin
with these approaches. Correspondingly, pharmacological treatment in children should be reserved for situations when other interventions have failed.
Drug treatments for insomnia are covered in greater detail in Table 7–5 of

Table 11–7.   Drug treatments for anxiety in children and adolescents

Drug by class	Suggested dosing, titration	Notes
	**Long-term strategies aimed at treatment of anxiety disorders**	
SSRIs and SNRIs		SSRIs and SNRIs are generally effective for the treatment of anxiety disorders in children and adolescents.
		Specific FDA indications vary from one drug to another; in practice, drugs are selected on the basis of side effects, access, and other distinguishing characteristics (see Chapter 3, Table 3–4). See Table 11–5 for dosing and titration information on specific drugs.
		Relative to the treatment of depression, in managing anxiety:
		• Treatment is often initiated at a lower dose.
		• Pace of titration is often slower.
		• Target dose is often higher.
Miscellaneous antidepressants (bupropion, mirtazapine)		Minimal data support the use of bupropion in anxiety disorders; it is not recommended for this purpose.
		A small amount of data suggests that mirtazapine may affect anxiety symptoms, but the strength of data strongly favors other agents.

Table 11–7.   Drug treatments for anxiety in children and adolescents *(continued)*

Drug by class	Suggested dosing, titration	Notes
Benzodiazepines	Short-term strategies aimed at rapid relief of symptoms	Effective anxiolytics, but use with caution in palliative care setting Cause sedation, confusion/delirium, falls, disinhibition Avoid short-half-life agents (e.g., alprazolam)
Lorazepam	6–13 years: 0.05 mg/kg (~0.125–1 mg) q 60 min prn anxiety 14–18 years: 0.25–2 mg q 60 min prn anxiety Max: ~10 mg/day (patient dependent)	Wide dose range; adjust to desired effect or side effect, then consider scheduled dose based on demand Half-life=12–14 hrs Despite long half-life, clinically often need to provide around-the-clock tid to qid dosing in severe anxiety Safer than clonazepam in liver failure Available routes: PO (tabs, liq), SL, SC, IM, IV
Clonazepam	6–13 years: 0.01–0.03 mg/kg/day, divided tid dosing (NTE 0.05 mg/kg/day) 14–18 years: 0.125–1 mg/dose Max: ~6 mg/day (patient dependent)	Wide dose range Half-life=30–40 hrs (despite this, many patients require tid dosing) Slower onset makes it less ideal for prn use Clonazepam 0.25 mg ≈ lorazepam 1 mg Available routes: PO (tabs, ODT)

Table 11–7. Drug treatments for anxiety in children and adolescents *(continued)*

Drug by class	Suggested dosing, titration	Notes
	Short-term strategies aimed at rapid relief of symptoms (continued)	
Other agents with "anxiolytic" properties		
		Expert opinion suggests that these can ameliorate anxiety and represent safer alternatives to benzodiazepines
		Use in the management of anxiety is off-label
Gabapentin	50–200 mg PO q 2 hrs prn anxiety	Wide dose range (NTE 3 doses or 600 mg/day)
	Max: ~3 doses in 24 hrs (patient dependent)	Effective in neuropathic pain
		Requires dose reduction in renal failure
		Available routes: PO (tabs, caps, liq)
Trazodone	6–13 years:	Off-label treatment of insomnia is most common use
	1.5–2 mg/kg/day; may titrate to 6 mg/kg/day	Adverse effects: sedation, restlessness, dry mouth, priapism (rare)
	14–18 years:	Wide dose range; adjust to desired effect/side effect, then consider scheduled dose based on demand
	start at 25–50 mg/day	Available routes: PO (tabs)
	Max: ~400 mg/day (patient dependent)	

Note. Dosing guidelines reflect a general strategy based on current drug references (Micromedex DRUGDEX 2014; Stahl 2014) and the clinical experience of the authors. Consult with local experts/resources for specific concerns (e.g., dosing strategies in incomplete responders, or dose adjustments in hepatic/renal insufficiency). caps=capsules; FDA=U.S. Food and Drug Administration; IM=intramuscular; IV=intravenous; liq=liquid; max=maximum; NTE=not to exceed; ODT=orally disintegrating tablet; PO=per oral; prn=as needed; q=every; qid=four times daily; SC=subcutaneous; SL=sublingual; SNRI=serotonin-norepinephrine reuptake inhibitor; SSRI=selective serotonin reuptake inhibitor; tabs=tablets; tid=three times daily.

Table 11–8.   Common causes of insomnia in children and adolescents

Cause	Examples/notes
Pain	Contributes to difficulty falling asleep and staying asleep. Analgesics (especially opiates and steroids) can worsen sleep. Severe pain creates a state of heightened arousal, which interferes with restful sleep (Raymond et al. 2001).
Respiratory problems	Cystic fibrosis: 40% of patients report sleep disturbances (Naqvi et al. 2008). Neuromuscular disorders (e.g., Duchenne muscular dystrophy; spinal muscle atrophy): Myopathies lead to respiratory muscle fatigue, especially later in the night (Bandla and Splaingard 2004). Obstructive sleep apnea Craniofacial deformities Severe scoliosis Obesity Central sleep apnea Nocturnal cough
Metabolic and genetic syndromes	Rett syndrome (Young et al. 2007) Angelman syndrome (Walz et al. 2005)
Structural brain lesions/ neurological disease	Especially those involving the brain stem, disruption to hypothalamic regulation of circadian rhythm, midline pathology, and blindness (Zucconi and Bruni 2001) Epilepsy (Kothare and Kaleyias 2010) Hydranencephaly
Cancer	Broadly, patients with cancer commonly have difficulties with sleep, especially as it relates to increased incidence of pain (Collins et al. 2000).
Terminal phase of illness	Up to 25% of children, broadly, at the end of life are found to have sleep disturbance (Drake et al. 2003; Theunissen et al. 2007).

Table 11–9. Nonpharmacological management of insomnia in pediatric palliative care

Intervention	Description
Environmental	Provide daytime exposure to natural light and graduated reduction in lighting exposure into the evening.
	Ensure that medications and treatments are not scheduled during sleeping hours.
	Provide a cool room temperature (but be mindful of patients with difficulty maintaining body temperature).
	Silence monitor alarms at night.
	Provide a comfortable bed.
	Encourage use of special pillow, blanket, or other transitional objects.
Behavioral	Maintain consistent evening routine (nighttime rituals, time of sleep, etc.), similar to that used at home if appropriate.
	Avoid painful or anxiety-producing procedures late in the day.
	Provide relaxation skills training.
	Provide hypnotherapy, including the use of specific guided imagery or soothing storytelling.
Special considerations	Exercise common sense with regard to setting limits around sleep in medically ill children.
	Consider behavioral interventions in the context of goals of care and prognosis.
	If nighttime is the only time when a child is alert, and prognosis is short, then families should consider relaxing expectations, to optimize quality of time together.

Chapter 7. Anticholinergic agents are usually avoided in this population due to concern for delirium. Nonetheless, in select cases, diphenhydramine or the antihistamine hydroxyzine may be used for insomnia in seriously ill children. Although it is not used for this purpose in adults, clonidine (0.05–0.3 mg PO qhs) may have a role in the treatment of insomnia in children (Owens 2009).

In addition, the benzodiazepine receptor agonists (e.g., zolpidem, zaleplon, eszopiclone) are generally avoided in children, but they may be used with caution and close monitoring. Recent data suggest a role for ramelteon, a melatonin receptor agonist, in the treatment of insomnia in some children, at doses ranging from 2 mg to 8 mg PO qhs (Asano et al. 2014; Kawabe et al. 2014). Caution is warranted, however, because these data are not from palliative care populations, and ramelteon has significant drug-drug interactions. When drug treatments are used for insomnia in children, lower initial doses should be selected, the lowest effective dose should be the target, and trials should have clear clinical goals and end points.

Delirium

As in adults, delirium in children with advanced medical illness is a common and serious condition, although the research base concerning delirium in this population is far less mature than that focused on adults. In one study of critically ill children, up to 30% were found to have delirium, and the condition was associated with longer ICU stays and a mortality rate of 20%–22% (Smith et al. 2013). Despite these findings, most institutions do not routinely screen for delirium in pediatric populations (Kudchadkar et al. 2014), and it is likely that the condition often goes unrecognized.

The assessment of delirium in pediatric populations can be quite challenging, particularly in very young children, in whom cognitive deficits may not be as evident as in adults. Hence, assessment must account for the child's level of cognitive development, and a careful clinical examination by a trained subspecialist, such as a child and adolescent psychiatrist, is considered the "gold standard" diagnostic approach. Several screening instruments can aid in identifying children likely to experience delirium. The Confusion Assessment Method (CAM), described in Chapter 5, "Delirium," has been adapted for children ages 6 months to 5 years (the Preschool CAM ICU), and for children over age 5 years (the Pediatric CAM ICU) (Smith et al. 2011). Similarly, the Cornell Assessment for Pediatric Delirium was developed for children ages 3 months through 21 years (Traube et al. 2014).

The approach to addressing delirium in children mirrors that used for adults, emphasizing providing support, ensuring safety, addressing the underlying cause, and using nonpharmacological and pharmacological treatments to ameliorate symptoms (see Chapter 5). With respect to nonpharmacological interventions, in pediatric palliative care parents can play an important role in helping to reduce symptoms: they should be involved in care to the extent possible, helping to provide familiar contact and a normal routine. Drug treatment in children, as in adults, relies on the use of antipsychotic medication for symptom management, as shown in Table 11–10. Haloperidol has been safely used in children with delirium (Brown et al. 1996), and its range of available routes (oral, intravenous, subcutaneous, intramuscular, and rectal) makes it particularly useful. Second-generation antipsychotics may be preferable in cases of hypoactive delirium (Turkel 2010), and in some circumstances benzodiazepines may play a role as well, as described in Chapter 5.

Conclusions and Key Points

- Skillful communication, appropriate to the child's developmental stage, is critical to the successful treatment of the child and adolescent palliative care patient.

- Children living with a life-limiting illness often have a more mature understanding of illness and death than healthy peers, but this should be explored carefully.

- The bidirectional relationship between physical and emotional symptoms is often particularly strong in pediatric populations; effective treatments need to comprehensively address total pain.

- Depression, anxiety, and insomnia are common in the pediatric palliative care population, and effective treatments exist, even in advanced stages of disease.

- Delirium causes significant distress and should be managed aggressively based on goals, likelihood of reversibility, and overall context of the patient.

Table 11–10.   Drug treatments for symptom management in delirium in children and adolescents

Drug by class	Suggested dosing, titration	Recommended prn interval (based on time to C_{max})	Recommended ATC interval (based on half-life)	Notes
Antipsychotics				Recommended in hyperactive delirium, reversible or irreversible. Data do not support efficacy of one agent over another; choose based on side effects, routes, cost, etc.
Haloperidol	1–3 years/10–20 kg: 0.1–0.4 mg/dose (max: 1 mg/day) 4–6 years/20–30 kg: 0.2–0.6 mg/dose (max: 2 mg/day) 7–10 years/30–40 kg: 0.3–0.8 mg/dose (max: 4 mg/day) 11–18 years/>40 kg: 0.4–1 mg/dose (max: 10 mg/day)	PO/PR: 60 min SC/IM: 30 min IV: 15 min	bid/tid	Max dose ~ patient dependent, based on tolerability, efficacy, goals Available routes: PO (tabs, liq), PR, SC, IM, IV

Table 11–10. Drug treatments for symptom management in delirium in children and adolescents *(continued)*

Drug by class	Suggested dosing, titration	Recommended prn interval (based on time to C_{max})	Recommended ATC interval (based on half-life)	Notes
Antipsychotics *(continued)*				
Olanzapine	7–10 years: 1.25–2.5 mg/dose (max: 5 mg/day) 11–18 years: 2.5–5 mg/dose (max: 10 mg/day)	PO: 60 min IM: 30 min	Daily/bid	Max dose ~ patient dependent, based on tolerability, efficacy, goals Available routes: PO (tabs, ODT), IM
Risperidone	4–6 years: 0.125–0.25 mg/dose (max: 1 mg/day) 7–13 years: 0.25 mg–0.5 mg/dose (max: 2 mg/day) 14–18 years: 0.25–1 mg/dose (max: 4 mg/day)	PO/PR: 60 min IM: 30 min	Daily/bid	Max dose ~ patient dependent, based on tolerability, efficacy, goals Available routes: PO (tabs, liq, ODT)

Table 11–10. Drug treatments for symptom management in delirium in children and adolescents *(continued)*

Drug by class	Suggested dosing, titration	Recommended prn interval (based on time to C_{max})	Recommended ATC interval (based on half-life)	Notes
Benzodiazepines				Recommended in 1) irreversible delirium, especially with signs of active dying; 2) alcohol or benzodiazepine withdrawal delirium; and 3) severe behavioral agitation. Patients receiving long-term benzodiazepine therapy (e.g., for anxiety) may be refractory to control of agitation with benzodiazepines.
Lorazepam	<12 years: 0.025–0.05 mg/kg/dose (~0.125–1 mg/dose) ≥12 years: 0.25–2 mg/dose	PO/PR: 60 min SC/IM: 30 min IV: 15 min	bid to qid	Max dose ~ patient dependent: <12 years: 4 mg/day ≥12 years: 10 mg/day Available routes: PO (tabs, liq), PR, SC, IM, IV In infants and young children, half-life is longer, thus requiring less-frequent dosing

Table 11–10. Drug treatments for symptom management in delirium in children and adolescents *(continued)*

Drug by class	Suggested dosing, titration	Recommended prn interval (based on time to C_{max})	Recommended ATC interval (based on half-life)	Notes
Benzodiazepines *(continued)*				
Midazolam	0.1–0.2 mg/kg SC loading dose Then repeat q 30 min prn for agitation Then give 25% of total dose needed to control symptoms as a continuous SC infusion	SC/IM: 30 min IV: 15 min	Continuous infusion	Max daily dose ~patient dependent based on efficacy, tolerability, goals Available routes: PO (liq), SC, IM, IV, IN, buccal

Note. No drug treatments have U.S. Food and Drug Administration approval for the management of delirium. Dosing guidelines reflect a general initial strategy based on the clinical experience of the authors and current drug references (Micromedex DRUGDEX 2014). Local experts and other resources should be consulted for specific concerns (e.g., dosing strategies in incomplete responders, or dose adjustments in hepatic/renal insufficiency). ATC=around the clock; bid=twice daily; C_{max}=maximum plasma concentration; IM=intramuscular; IV=intravenous; liq=liquid; ODT=orally disintegrating tablet; PO=per oral; PR=per rectum; prn=as needed; q=every; qid=four times daily; SC=subcutaneous; tabs=tablets; tid=three times daily.

References

Asano M, Ishitobi M, Kosaka H, et al: Ramelteon monotherapy for insomnia and impulsive behavior in high-functioning autistic disorder. J Clin Psychopharmacol 34(3):402–403, 2014 24717259

Bandla H, Splaingard M: Sleep problems in children with common medical disorders. Pediatr Clin North Am 51(1):203–227, viii, 2004 15008590

Beale EA, Baile WF, Aaron J: Silence is not golden: communicating with children dying from cancer. J Clin Oncol 23(15):3629–3631, 2005 15908676

Brown RL, Henke A, Greenhalgh DG, et al: The use of haloperidol in the agitated, critically ill pediatric patient with burns. J Burn Care Rehabil 17(1):34–38, 1996 8808357

Chavira DA, Garland AF, Daley S, et al: The impact of medical comorbidity on mental health and functional health outcomes among children with anxiety disorders. J Dev Behav Pediatr 29(5):394–402, 2008 18714205

Collins JJ, Byrnes ME, Dunkel IJ, et al: The measurement of symptoms in children with cancer. J Pain Symptom Manage 19(5):363–377, 2000 10869877

Collins JJ, Devine TD, Dick GS, et al: The measurement of symptoms in young children with cancer: the validation of the Memorial Symptom Assessment Scale in children aged 7–12. J Pain Symptom Manage 23(1):10–16, 2002 11779663

Drake R, Frost J, Collins JJ: The symptoms of dying children. J Pain Symptom Manage 26(1):594–603, 2003 12850642

Fosson A, deQuan MM: Reassuring and talking with hospitalized children. Child Health Care 13(1):37–44, 1984 10267187

Hamilton BE, Hoyert DL, Martin JA, et al: Annual summary of vital statistics: 2010–2011. Pediatrics 131(3):548–558, 2013 23400611

Himelstein BP, Hilden JM, Boldt AM, et al: Pediatric palliative care. N Engl J Med 350(17):1752–1762, 2004 15103002

Hirsh CD, Friebert S: Primary pediatric palliative care: psychological and social support for children and families. Pediatr Rev 35(9):390–395, 2014 25183774

Kawabe K, Horiuchi F, Oka Y, et al: The melatonin receptor agonist ramelteon effectively treats insomnia and behavioral symptoms in autistic disorder. Case Report Psychiatry 2014:561071, 2014 24955274

Kothare SV, Kaleyias J: Sleep and epilepsy in children and adolescents. Sleep Med 11(7):674–685, 2010 20620102

Kreicbergs U, Valdimarsdóttir U, Onelöv E, et al: Talking about death with children who have severe malignant disease. N Engl J Med 351(12):1175–1186, 2004 15371575

Kreitler S, Oppenheim D, Segey-Shoham E: Fantasy, art therapies, humor and pets as psychosocial means of intervention, in Psychosocial Aspects of Pediatric Oncology. Edited by Kreitler S, Weyl Ben Arush M. Hoboken, NJ, Wiley, 2004, pp 351–388

Kudchadkar SR, Yaster M, Punjabi NM: Sedation, sleep promotion, and delirium screening practices in the care of mechanically ventilated children: a wake-up call for the pediatric critical care community. Crit Care Med 42(7):1592–1600, 2014 24717461

Lambert V, Glacken M, McCarron M: "Visible-ness": the nature of communication for children admitted to a specialist children's hospital in the Republic of Ireland. J Clin Nurs 17(23):3092–3102, 2008 19012779

Levetown M; American Academy of Pediatrics Committee on Bioethics: Communicating with children and families: from everyday interactions to skill in conveying distressing information. Pediatrics 121(5):e1441–e1460, 2008 18450887

Lewin DS, Dahl RE: Importance of sleep in the management of pediatric pain. J Dev Behav Pediatr 20(4):244–252, 1999 10475599

Lieverse R, Van Someren EJ, Nielen MM, et al: Bright light treatment in elderly patients with nonseasonal major depressive disorder: a randomized placebo-controlled trial. Arch Gen Psychiatry 68(1):61–70, 2011 21199966

March JS, Silva S, Petrycki S, et al: The Treatment for Adolescents With Depression Study (TADS): long-term effectiveness and safety outcomes. Arch Gen Psychiatry 64(10):1132–1143, 2007 17909125

Micromedex DRUGDEX (Internet database). Ann Arbor, MI, Truven Health Analytics, 2014. Available at: www.micromedexsolutions.com. Subscription required to view.

Naqvi SK, Sotelo C, Murry L, et al: Sleep architecture in children and adolescents with cystic fibrosis and the association with severity of lung disease. Sleep Breath 12(1):77–83, 2008 17610099

Owens JA: Pharmacotherapy of pediatric insomnia. J Am Acad Child Adolesc Psychiatry 48(2):99–107, 2009 20040822

Owens JA, Dalzell V: Use of the "BEARS" sleep screening tool in a pediatric residents' continuity clinic: a pilot study. Sleep Med 6(1):63–69, 2005 15680298

Pao M, Weiner L: Psychological symptoms, in Textbook of Interdisciplinary Pediatric Palliative Care. Edited by Wolfe J, Hinds PS, Sourkes BM. Philadelphia, PA, Elsevier/Saunders, 2011, pp 229–238

Powers SW: Empirically supported treatments in pediatric psychology: procedure-related pain. J Pediatr Psychol 24(2):131–145, 1999 10361392

Quill TE, Bower K, Holloway RG, et al: Primer of Palliative Care, 6th Edition. Glenview, IL, American Academy of Hospice and Palliative Medicine, 2014

Raymond I, Nielsen TA, Lavigne G, et al: Quality of sleep and its daily relationship to pain intensity in hospitalized adult burn patients. Pain 92(3):381–388, 2001 11376911

Schonfeld DJ: Talking with children about death. J Pediatr Health Care 7(6):269–274, 1993 8106926

Smith HA, Boyd J, Fuchs DC, et al: Diagnosing delirium in critically ill children: validity and reliability of the Pediatric Confusion Assessment Method for the Intensive Care Unit. Crit Care Med 39(1):150–157, 2011 20959783

Smith HA, Berutti T, Brink E, et al: Pediatric critical care perceptions on analgesia, sedation, and delirium. Semin Respir Crit Care Med 34(2):244–261, 2013 23716315

Spirito A, Kazak AE: Effective and Emerging Treatments in Pediatric Psychology. New York, Oxford University Press, 2006

Stahl SM: Essential Psychopharmacology: The Prescriber's Guide. Cambridge, UK, Cambridge University Press, 2014

Swedo SE, Allen AJ, Glod CA, et al: A controlled trial of light therapy for the treatment of pediatric seasonal affective disorder. J Am Acad Child Adolesc Psychiatry 36(6):816–821, 1997 9183137

Theunissen JM, Hoogerbrugge PM, van Achterberg T, et al: Symptoms in the palliative phase of children with cancer. Pediatr Blood Cancer 49(2):160–165, 2007 16972239

Traube C, Silver G, Kearney J, et al: Cornell Assessment of Pediatric Delirium: a valid, rapid, observational tool for screening delirium in the PICU*. Crit Care Med 42(3):656–663, 2014 24145848

Turkel SB: Delirium, in Textbook of Pediatric Psychosomatic Medicine. Edited by Shaw RJ, DeMaso DR. Washington, DC, American Psychiatric Publishing, 2010, pp 63–25

Walz NC, Beebe D, Byars K: Sleep in individuals with Angelman syndrome: parent perceptions of patterns and problems. Am J Ment Retard 110(4):243–252, 2005 15941362

Wolfe J, Hinds PS, Sourkes BM (eds): Textbook of Interdisciplinary Pediatric Palliative Care. Philadelphia, PA, Elsevier/Saunders, 2011

Young D, Nagarajan L, de Klerk N, et al: Sleep problems in Rett syndrome. Brain Dev 29(10):609–616, 2007 17531413

Zucconi M, Bruni O: Sleep disorders in children with neurologic diseases. Semin Pediatr Neurol 8(4):258–275, 2001 11768788

Additional Resources

Aldridge J, Sourkes BM: The psychological impact of life-limiting conditions on the child, in Oxford Textbook of Palliative Care for Children, 2nd Edition. Edited by Goldman A, Hain R, Liben S. New York, Oxford University Press, 2012, pp 78–89

Brown MR, Sourkes B: Psychotherapy in pediatric palliative care. Child Adolesc Psychiatr Clin N Am 15(3):585–596, 2006

Friebert S, Bower KA, Lookabough B: UNIPAC 8: Caring for Pediatric Patients UNIPAC Self Study Program, 4th Edition. Edited by Storey CP Jr. Glenview, IL, American Academy of Hospice and Palliative Medicine, 2012. Available at: http://www.aahpm.org/resources/default/unipac-4th-edition.html. Accessed July 30, 2015.

ICU Delirium and Cognitive Impairment Study Group. Web site at: http://icu-delirium.org.

Knapp C, Madden V, Button D, et al: Partnerships between pediatric palliative care and psychiatry. Pediatr Clin North Am 58(4):1025–1039, 2011

Muriel AC, McCulloch R, Hammel JF: Depression, anxiety, and delirium, in Oxford Textbook of Palliative Care for Children, 2nd Edition. Edited by Goldman A, Hain R, Liben S. New York, Oxford University Press, 2012, pp 309–318

Sourkes BM, Wolfe J: The child and adolescent in palliative care, in Handbook of Psychiatry in Palliative Medicine, 2nd Edition. Edited by Chochinov HM, Breitbart W. New York, Oxford University Press, 2009, pp 531–543

Stuber ML, Bursch B: Psychiatric care of the terminally ill child, in Handbook of Psychiatry in Palliative Medicine, 2nd Edition. Edited by Chochinov HM, Breitbart W. New York, Oxford University Press, 2009, pp 519–530

Index

*Page numbers printed in **boldface** type refer to tables or figures.*

.

CPSIA information can be obtained
at www.ICGtesting.com
Printed in the USA
LVOW04s1656050316

477897LV00002B/2/P

9 781585 624768